WORLD HEALTH
ORGANIZATION

ORGANISATION MONDIALE
DE LA SANTÉ

WHO/Mal/174 Rev. 1
WHO/HS/58 Rev. 1
2 September 1957

ENGLISH ONLY

STATISTICAL METHODOLOGY

IN

MALARIA WORK

by

Satya Swaroop
Chief, Statistical Studies Section
World Health Organization

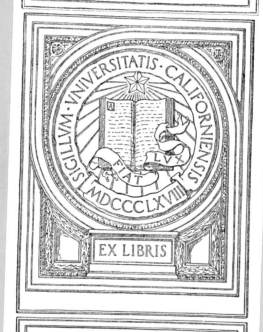

WORLD HEALTH
ORGANIZATION

ORGANISATION MONDIALE
DE LA SANTÉ

WHO/Mal/174 Rev.1
WHO/HS/58 Rev.1
2 September 1957

ENGLISH ONLY

STATISTICAL METHODOLOGY

IN

MALARIA WORK

by

Satya Swaroop
Chief, Statistical Studies Section
World Health Organization

CONTENTS

Page

APPENDICES

LIST OF TABLES

LIST OF FIGURES

STATISTICAL METHODOLOGY IN MALARIA WORK

1.   INTRODUCTION

Important advances are being made in malariology.   New methods for cure, control, or eradication of the disease are put forward from time to time, but sometimes exaggerated claims appear in the press for discoveries which ultimately prove either to be of no scientific value or to have no advantage over other methods. On the other hand, sometimes a method of definite utility may escape recognition because inadequately planned experiments conducted to test its value might, under certain circumstances, have yielded inconsistent results.   For these reasons, it is now customary, when a new theory or method is put forward, to subject it to properly planned tests, under circumstances in which its validity is claimed, so as to obtain conclusive evidence.

The scientific method of study demands objectivity of approach, i.e. it should be kept independent of the personal bias or subjective judgement of the worker. Objectivity of approach is difficult to achieve without recourse to the careful recording of numerical observations.   Lord Kelvin truly said that:

> "When you can measure what you are speaking about and express it in numbers, you know something about it, but when you cannot measure it, when you cannot express it in numbers, your knowledge is of a meagre and unsatisfactory kind."

Francis Galton expressed the same idea differently when he said that:

> "General impressions are never to be trusted.   Unfortunately, when they are of long standing they become fixed rules of life and assume a prescriptive right not to be questioned.   Consequently, those who are not accustomed to original enquiry entertain a hatred and a horror of statistics.   They cannot endure the idea of submitting their sacred impressions to coldblooded verification.   But it is the triumph of scientific man to rise superior to such superstitions, to desire tests by which the value of their beliefs may be ascertained and to feel sufficiently masters of themselves to discard contemptuously whatever may be found untrue."

If the data collected by malariologists were as simple as are generally recorded in such exact sciences as physics or astronomy, then perhaps the need for statistical methodology may not have been fully appreciated. But while physicists and astronomers deal with inanimate objects, a malariologist has to consider data relating at once to the interaction of three living populations of the animal kingdom, viz. the man, the arthropod insect and the protozoan malaria parasite. Further, each of these may affect and be affected by environmental and other known and unknown factors. We are thus concerned with data which relate not only to highly variable beings but are also affected by a multiplicity of factors producing this variability. The study of malaria, therefore, is complex in the extreme, and more so than any other disease we know. Proper methods of analysing and interpreting such data are therefore needed. Otherwise, there may be a temptation for a worker to lay undue emphasis on some selected aspect of variability and arrive at conclusions which are not justified. Modern statistical methods are designed especially to take account of numerical data which are affected to a marked degree by a multiplicity of causes. This relatively new science of statistical methodology not only provides useful methods of dealing with data arising from the influence of highly variable factors, it also opens up a new means of bringing about uniformity in the analysis of, and more so in the conclusions arrived at from, the same data by different workers. For these reasons, the use of modern statistical methods in connexion with the planning of field trials or demonstration projects, and in the subsequent interpretation and evaluation of results, has now become a recognized procedure for the scientific study of biological phenomena. Indeed it is the essence of scientific work in malaria that facts and figures from each individual locality are carefully recorded, local conditions affecting malaria are narrated and finally the data are subjected to standard statistical methods and techniques, so that workers in any other part of the world can repeat the observations and arrive at comparable results.

The term "statistics" is sometimes understood to connote merely the mass of numerical information collected and arranged in rows and columns of a table. Thus, the term "malaria statistics" may be understood to mean merely the data collected or arising in connexion with malaria work. It is however necessary to point out that the term "statistics" also connotes a methodology - a scientific technique - for dealing with such data. More specifically it may be called "statistical methodology".

Broadly stated it is a science dealing with:

1.   the proper collection of data, which includes:

1.1   the development of standard definitions, classification and recording procedures;

1.2   proper planning or designing and conduct of laboratory experiments, surveys, field trials, or research projects;

1.3   the scrutiny of data for accuracy, completeness and adequacy;

2.   analysis and interpretation of data, including:

2.1   the sorting and classification of data into suitable classes or groups and preparation of tables;

2.2   the estimation of necessary statistical indices and constants;

2.3   the statistical assessment of the significance of main findings or conclusions;

3.   the presentation of data and results in the form of text, tables and diagrams.

Of these, the items 1.2 and 2.3 viz. the planning of experiments, surveys, or field trials and the analysis of data, especially by the application of modern statistical techniques for the assessment of the significance of results, are highly specialized fields.

All the above aspects are of course well discussed in many excellent textbooks on the subject. It would therefore be futile to prepare a separate book for malaria workers. All the same, an initiation of malaria workers into the statistical method of approach seems necessary especially because of the wide extension of malaria projects in different parts of the world, and also for fear lest, without proper use of this approach, much of the valuable scientific data may lie unused or may be lost. Therefore, guided by past experience, this document has been prepared to indicate to malaria workers some of the basic statistical principles that should constantly be kept in mind and to explain how the application of recommended statistical procedures as well as collaboration with the statistician may help in planning, executing and evaluating the projects on sounder scientific lines. For reasons of brevity what has been attempted is only an introduction to usable statistical techniques in malaria work.

This document, therefore, has merely the character and purpose of general "notes" to facilitate the work of field malaria workers, not pretending in any way to be a substitute for textbooks on statistical methodology or for specialized papers on malariometry. Those who may like to study specific aspects in greater detail will find appropriate references mentioned in the text. Neither is it intended that this document should replace collaboration with the statistician. On the contrary, it is hoped that a study of this document will reveal some of the advantages which expert handling of the statistical aspect of malaria work can provide.

Like any other scientific technique, statistical methodology is also designed to provide uniformity in the method of handling data, thus bringing about objectivity and comparability in the analysis, interpretation and presentation of results. In this connexion important advances have already been made in malariometry by the publication by WHO of the monograph on "Malaria Terminology" (Covell et al., 1953), intended to standardize the definitions of terms including malariometric indices, as well as by the preparation of WHO document MAL/DEM Rev.1 of December 1951.

This document may be similarly regarded as providing hints for securing uniformity in the statistical aspects of malaria work. The need for such a document to supplement the other two documents and to initiate malaria workers into statistical ways of thinking has long been felt and has now become increasingly important with the wide extension of malaria projects in different parts of the world. It is hoped that an understanding of the role that statistical methodology can play in malaria work will make it possible for much valuable scientific data to be properly used and made available to other workers.

The contents of this document have been so arranged that the reader is first acquainted with a few of the simple statistical concepts and techniques and the terminology used in modern statistical methodology. By means of examples relating to malaria, an explanation is given of the manner in which the statistician usually proceeds to analyse the data, the arguments he uses for assessing the statistical significance of results and the various estimates, together with their errors, which he deduces. Almost all the numerical examples given in this document are derived from literature or reports on malaria. Brief reference is also made to statistical information collected by national statistical services which malaria workers may find useful.

These basic data and the statistical methods of presentation and assessment of results having been discussed, the next section is devoted to some of the common statistical problems malaria workers are known to have had to face in connexion with the planning, execution and evaluation of their projects. In order to facilitate the adoption of some of the recommended statistical procedures, some tables and charts are included from which the results can be read merely at a glance, i.e. without having to undertake any complicated calculations.

Some malariologists may entertain a fear of the term 'statistics' inasmuch as it may seem to them to require a knowledge of higher mathematics. They may rest assured that many mathematicians also may not know much about statistical techniques; they too have to learn this science as a separate discipline. Nor can statistics be regarded as simple arithmetic. Even though arithmetical calculations are needed for the application of statistical methodology at various stages, so many simplifications have been introduced that by means of ready-reckoning tables, a slide rule or preferably a calculating machine, recourse to laborious computational work is almost obviated. If the usefulness of statistical methodology can be appreciated, which indeed is the main object of this document, it should open the way for more fruitful collaboration with the statistician to whom all the routine computation work could be entrusted.

This document developed in response to requests received from malaria workers during the past few years for statistical assistance in their work. A series of notes on statistical methodology were prepared from time to time. In May 1956 the preparation of these notes was sufficiently well advanced to put them together in a document entitled "Statistical Notes for Malaria Workers" (WHO/Mal/174 or WHO/HS/58), of which mimeographed copies were made available to interested malaria and health statistics workers. Many helpful suggestions were made for its improvement and revision, and these are incorporated in the present document. Thus while some portions considered too advanced have been deleted, a few notable additions are in respect of vital and health statistics rates, the estimation of LD_{50} in connexion with studies on the development of anopheline resistance to insecticides, and certain statistical problems relating to malaria eradication.   In the preparation of both the original document and the present revision, the author received guidance and encouragement from Drs E. J. Pampana (Director, Malaria Eradication), Y. Biraud (Director, Division of Epidemiological and Health Statistical Services) and M. Pascua (formerly Director-Consultant, Health Statistics), to whom grateful acknowledgement is made, as also to Mr K. Uemura of the Statistical Studies Section and Ir D. Sonti, both of whom have rendered valuable assistance in the preparation of this document.   Among those who have assisted with valuable comments in the revision of this document, the author wishes in particular to thank Drs L. J. Bruce-Chwatt, G. Grammiccia, B. Weeks and J. de Zulueta.

2. STATISTICAL METHODS FOR MALARIA WORKERS

2.1 Collection of Data

In malaria work data may be collected from various sources such as field surveys or trials, demonstration projects, laboratory examinations or from previously collected records or reports. From whatever source or experience they are derived, the findings are dependable only to the extent that the data upon which they are based are accurate, comparable, and representative of the experience they describe. It is necessary at the very start, therefore, to scrutinize the data for adequacy, completeness and accuracy. Various sources of bias and error which can enter into the collection of information should be recognized and avoided, as for instance, those arising through lack of understanding of the definitions of terms used, inaccuracies in the measuring instruments, bias of the observer, or sheer carelessness. The limitations of the data must therefore be fully recognized, various sources of error noted, accounted for and, as far as possible, eliminated.

Sometimes there is a tendency to embark on an over-ambitious programme for the collection of information. In the interests of economy and efficiency, as far as possible, only such data need be recorded as are to be put to use in subsequent analysis and understanding of the problem under study. As early as 1832, Quetelet, the Belgian statistician, offered the following four precepts which, if kept in mind, should enhance the quality of the numerical information collected:

"(1) Have no preconceived ideas. Be unbiased. Attack your problem with an open mind.

(2) Don't reject contrary values. Eliminate possible errors then seek verification of the contrary values. Face the facts you find.

(3) Note all possible causes. Test them or control them.

(4) Compare data that are comparable. Accurate comparisons can be made only between similar things and over short periods of time. Data drawn from unlike sources may lead to false interpretations."

2.2 Classification

During the course of malaria survey or experimental work a large volume of
statistical information relating to an overwhelming mass of detail may be accumulated.
It is not easy for the human mind to grasp fully all the salient and significant
features without further analysis.   The first necessity in statistical analysis
therefore is to summarize the data in convenient form so as to bring out the main
features.   This is achieved by the process of classification, in which items which
need not be distinguished from each other are put together in groups, thus producing
what in statistical terminology are called "grouped data".   The underlying idea is
at first to decide what factors should form the basis of the study, and then to
proceed to arrange each individual item of information in such a way that "like is
associated with like", and that facts which relate to different characteristics are
arranged in separate categories.   Such a process of "classification", i.e. arranging
the data into well-defined categories, and the next step of "tabulation", i.e.
presentation of classified data in an orderly and systematic form in tables, help
considerably to elucidate the problems under consideration.

Frequently the categories into which data should be sorted out or classified
are suggested by the problem itself.   Thus, if we are interested in studying sex
differences in the spleen rate, the first step would be to classify the children
examined into males and females.   Next, we would classify the children in each sex
group separately according to whether they showed enlargement of spleen or not.
If we are interested in studying the distribution of spleen size, we will naturally
classify children in any age-group by spleen size, namely: 0, 1, 2, 3, 4, and 5
respectively, as stipulated by the WHO Drafting Committee on Malaria Terminology
(Covell et al., 1953, page 38).

It may be stated that for the majority of statistical measurements commonly made,
certain standard classifications are now in common use, many of which have in recent
years been recommended or agreed upon at the international level.   It is necessary to
adhere to the classifications so recommended.   In the absence of any such recommendation
it is advisable to follow the classifications set out in standard government
publications of the country concerned.   Adherence to the commonly accepted
classifications serves to provide comparability of data with those from other countries,
regions or projects.   Some examples of the standard classifications recommended are
the following.

For the purpose of malaria work, the WHO Drafting Committee on Malaria Terminology (Covell et al., 1953, page 30) have recommended the following age-groupings:

Group	Description
0-11 months	Infants, babies
12-23 months	Children from one year to under two years of age
2- 4 years	"Toddlers", pre-school children
5- 9 years	Juveniles
10-14 years	Adolescents
15-19 years	Young adults
20 years and over	Adults

It may be explained that the age-group "0-11 months" read as "zero through 11 months"
will include all under 12 months of age.   A child of 12 months but under 24 months
will be classified in the next age-group "12-23 months".

The above age-groups are used for special reasons for classifying spleen and
blood examination data.   But for the purpose of tabulating national mortality
statistics by cause of death, WHO has recommended in its International Regulations
No. I the adoption of the following age classification.

Article 6 of Additional Regulations, amending WHO Regulations No. I of 1948
states that:

"In publishing statistics of causes of death by age one of the following
age-groupings shall be used:

(a) for general purposes:

(i)   under 1 year, single years to 4 years inclusive, five-year
groups from 5 to 84 years, 85 years and over;

(ii) under 1 year, 1-4 years, 5-14 years, 15-24 years, 25-44 years,
45-64 years, 65-74 years, 75 years and over;

(iii) under 1 year, 1-14 years, 15-44 years, 45-64 years, 65 years
and over;

(b)　for special statistics of infant mortality:

(i)　by single days for the first week of life (under 1 day, 1, 2, 3, 4, 5, 6 days), 7-13 days, 14-20 days, 21-27 days, 28 days up to but not including 2 months, by single month of life from 2 months to 1 year (2, 3, 4, ... 11 months);

(ii)　under 7 days, 7-27 days, 28 days up to but not including 3 months, 3-5 months, 6-11 months;

(iii)　under 28 days, 28 days to 11 months inclusive.

If age-groupings are published in greater detail than in one of the groupings specified above, they shall be so arranged as to allow condensation into one of these groupings."

While specifying age-groups there is the possibility of ambiguity because the age in years may happen to be recorded either as the age at the last birthday, the age at the nearest birthday, or the age at the next birthday. Such ambiguity can be avoided if the exact age in years, months, etc. is first worked out from the date of birth, or estimated. In the classifications suggested above it is to be noted that any given age figure includes persons from that age to just under the age specifying the beginning of the next class interval.

For the purpose of classifying causes of death with a view to securing international comparability, WHO has recommended (WHO Regulations No. I) that all countries follow the International Statistical Classification of Diseases, Injuries, and Causes of Death as set out in the Manual, Volume I (WHO 1957). An alphabetical index of the various causes of death has been published as Volume II to facilitate the selection of the appropriate code number of each cause. The Detailed List is given in three-digit categories, with a further tabular list of inclusions in four-digit sub-categories. Special shorter lists for the tabulation of causes of death of 150 causes (Intermediate List A) and 50 causes (Abbreviated List B), have also been suggested. This Manual also prescribes a form for the medical certification of causes of death, to enable the underlying cause of death to be specified by the physician, and to facilitate the tabulation of the underlying cause of death for statistical purposes. Rules and instructions for dealing with joint causes of death are also given.

In many cases, however, the data themselves or the problem under study may not suggest a clear-cut method of classification. The problem occurs if, for instance, we wish to classify children according to weight, height, etc. The question then is: how many classes should we have? The number of classes would depend on the nature of the data, but as a practical rule, if the number of measurements is fairly large it is advisable to choose between 10 to 20 groups. Too many classes would in fact defeat the very purpose of classification, producing irregularities in the tabulated figures. On the other hand, too few classes will tend to group in each class dissimilar items of information, and may obscure the essential differences. As a general rule the larger the number of observations the finer should be the classification.

2.3 Use of Punched Cards for Recording Project Data

In the carrying out of malaria surveys, data may have to be recorded separately for individual households or for individual persons examined for spleen or malaria parasites, so as to study improvements with the progress of time. Such information may have to be recorded on hundreds or thousands of individuals, sometimes covering a large number of items of information in respect of each. For instance, in connexion with spleen and parasite examinations alone we shall need to record, in respect of each individual, the name (possibly also the father's name, name of village or locality, for the purpose of identification), sex, age, housing conditions, the size of the spleen at periodic intervals, duration of residence in the locality, and the results of blood examinations carried out from time to time, etc. Appropriate pro forma have been suggested in WHO document MAL/DEM Rev.1. When information is collected on such a large number of items for a very large number of individuals, the subsequent analysis of the data may involve an enormous amount of clerical work especially if the interrelationship of two or more factors has to be studied. The compilation of new tables each time then becomes a colossal task unless some devices are adopted to reduce this work. In this connexion the use of registers or loose sheets of paper, in which information is recorded in different rows or columns for a number of individuals, is generally to be deprecated. On the other hand, the use of punched cards as suggested below, and of mechanical systems for sorting and tabulating can result in the most remarkable saving of time and is recommended. The use of a separate card for each individual is indeed necessary for recording data if a mass of information has to be properly handled and analysed.

2.3.1   Marginally punched cards

The simplest and the most commonly employed card is that known as the Paramount
System card, variously named as Cope-Chat, Paramount, or McBee cards.   The special
feature of such a card, made of light cardboard, is that it has perforations along
one or more of its edges.   Each hole represents an item of information and is
identified by either a numbered or lettered code.   When the required information
has been entered on the card the relevant hole is slotted with a pair of nippers
similar to ticket collectors' nippers.   Slotting consists of making the closed holes
into open "V" shaped slots.

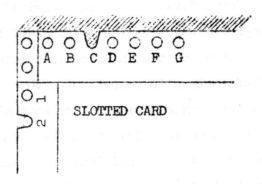

When a needle is inserted through a batch of cards and the batch is raised, those cards
which have been slotted at the needled position will fall away.   A sample card for
use by WHO malaria teams is reproduced here for purposes solely of illustration (Fig. 1).
A different card may be designed to fulfil the peculiar needs of each project.
For instance, Boyd (1949) has designed similar marginally punched cards to serve as
(a) malaria epidemiological record, (b) captured adult anophelines record, and
(c) anopheline breeding place record.   The designing of suitable cards is easy once
the principles of the system are understood.   In the body of this card space has
been provided for recording by hand the desired information, especially that which
has no subsequent statistical value (the names of the person and of the head of the

FIG. 1 AN EXAMPLE OF MARGINAL PUNCH CARD USED IN MALARIA SURVEY.

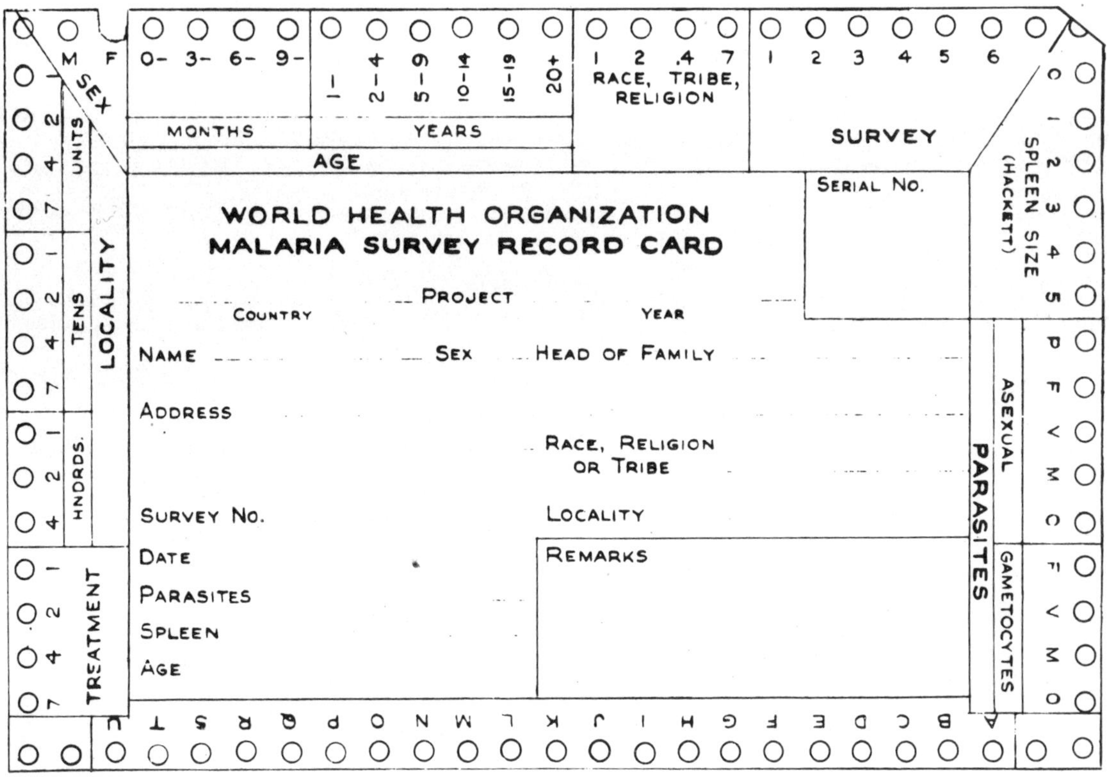

Fig. 2 Handling of marginally punched cards

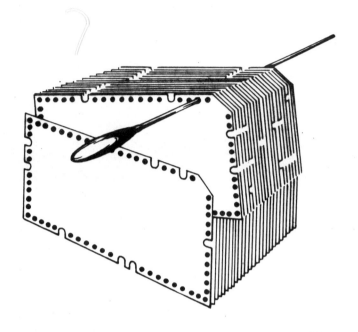

WHO 7317

family, address, etc.) as well as other data. In fact the body of the card can be printed and used as an ordinary record card. Information can be dictated in the field itself to a clerk. The reverse side of the card can also be used for the same purpose. It will be observed that each perforation has some specific information shown against it: for instance, the two holes to record sex at the left-hand side of the top edge are marked M and F to designate male or female.

The upper right-hand corner of the card is clipped off to facilitate stacking; a disarranged card then shows up by an uncut protruding corner. If the cards are properly stacked and a needle is passed through the hole marked F (denoting female), the whole stack can be lifted on it, but if a hole has been opened out by clipping off, as in Fig. 2, the card will fall off when lifted by the needle passed through "F" hole. A simple hand punching machine is available for opening out the holes in this manner. Thus, if we have a pack of 1000 or more cards and a long needle is inserted so as to pass through the hole denoting F, and the whole pack is then lifted and gently shaken, what would happen is that those cards in which the hole is open (cards of female individuals), will drop off, thus separating mechanically the entire pack into males and females. In the same manner, by passing the needle through the six holes marked for spleen size, the individuals can be subdivided according to the size of the spleen as well as by sex. Cards thus separated can then be counted, or what is more convenient, may be weighed, and their number estimated, provided we use a balance sensitive enough to detect the weight of a single card. When sorting, the most satisfactory results are obtained by taking a convenient handfull of cards and using the free hand to control the cards which fall out. Selection is quick and accurate. Approximately one thousand cards can be needled through any one position in one minute.

2.3.1.1 Coding

A variety of codes are available according to the requirements of the case. If high numbers are necessary running into tens of thousands, and the size of the card must be kept down, one of the condensed codes will answer the purpose. In addition to numerical codes, individual holes may have printed against them initials or letters. The following are a few illustrations of codes used. The "V's" shown represent slotted holes.

0 - 9 Code

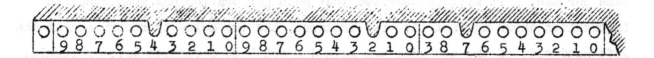

Punched for 427

The above illustrates the simplest form of numerical coding, called straight coding. A series of ten holes is allotted for units, tens, hundreds, thousands, until the desired limit is reached, each series bearing numbers 0 to 9 under the respective holes. A complete numerical sequence is thus obtained with a minimum amount of slotting.

7,4,2,1 Code

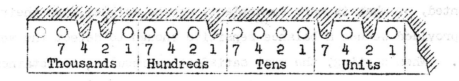

Punched for 6109

When the amount of coding to be done is such that a large card would be required, the size of the card can be greatly reduced by adopting the code shown above.

```
Slot 1 . . . . . . . . . = 1      Slot 4 and 2 . . . . . = 6
 "   2 . . . . . . . . . = 2       "   7 . . . . . . . . = 7
 "   2 and 1 . . . . . . = 3       "   7 and 1 . . . . . = 8
 "   4 . . . . . . . . . = 4       "   7 and 2 . . . . . = 9
 "   4 and 1 . . . . . . = 5      No slotting . . . . . = 0
```

The digits 7,4,2,1 are chosen because by opening out either only one or at the most two holes any number from 1 to 9 may be recorded.

In this code a hole for nought is not provided. Where a nought appears in the number to be coded, by not slotting any hole in this particular field or section, the nought is carried away on the needle after sorting the other numbers.

The method of recording numerical data on such cards (condensed code) will be clear from an explanation of how the code number of the locality can be punched, in Fig. 1. The four holes marked 1, 2, 4 and 7 are reserved for the units' space, another set of similarly marked four holes for the tenth space and three for the digit in the hundredth place appear on the left-hand side of the card as shown below.

```
┌─────────────────────────────────────────┐
│  ᴜ   ᴜ        ᴜ   ᴜ                       │
│ 0   0  0  0  0   0  0  0  0   0  0        │
├─────────────────────────────────────────┤
│  4  2  1  7  4  2  1  7  4   2  1         │
├─────────────────────────────────────────┤
│  Hundreds   Tens      Units               │
├─────────────────────────────────────────┤
│  Serial number of the locality            │
└─────────────────────────────────────────┘
```

Let us suppose the serial number or code number of the village is 235. The hole marked 2 is opened out in the hundredth place. Two holes marked 1 and 2 are opened out in the tenth place to denote 2 + 1 or 3: two holes marked 4 and 1 are similarly opened out in the units' space to denote the digit 4 + 1 or 5.

Other codes. Many other coding arrangements are available. Cards can be punched for numerical, alphabetical, geographic, chronological, direct or any coding or sorting method desired. An example of an alphabetical code is given below showing the punching for letter "N".

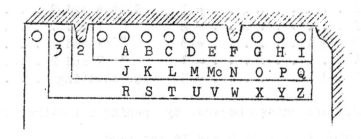

Punched for the initial letter 'N'

The perforations and printing on these cards can be designed to suit any special type of survey by the commercial firm which also supplies, in addition to such printed cards, a simple machine for punching and a needle for sorting purposes. Such cards are available in various sizes depending on the nature of the survey. The preparation of a punched card is in fact equivalent to posting of information in a register for original entry, but is much quicker, more accurate, and considerably less expensive. Much time is saved if the information can be directly punched on to these cards to save unnecessary writing by the field staff.

Such cards can be obtained in different colours so that each colour can denote a separate survey, or place or year of study, etc.

When alterations are to be made to the information punched on the card, or if a hole has been wrongly punched, it is not necessary to make out a fresh card. Patches are supplied for sticking over any slotted portions which are to be cancelled.

2.3.2 Electrical devices for punching, sorting and tabulation

The use of marginally perforated cards is advisable when the number of individuals is not likely to exceed a few thousand. For a more voluminous set of data another type of card is used in which punched holes are made in the body of the card to facilitate mechanical sorting and counting by electric machines. Such machines are available nowadays in most of the large towns. It is therefore advisable to make arrangements with an electrically operated punch card installation in some nearby office, so that the sorting and counting can be done electrically. Such equipment is installed by the IBM of USA, Powers Samas of UK, and British Remington or the British Tabulating Machine Company, etc. In this system also, information collected in respect of each individual is conveyed by means of punched holes to specially designed cards. For this purpose, the cards are passed through a punching machine by means of which holes are perforated in appropriate places, each perforation denoting a special item of coded information. An expert operator can punch about 5000 holes in an hour. The initial punching stage is the only operation into which the human element enters, and with the help of verifying machines a remarkable degree of accuracy can be assured. Thereafter the sorting or classifying of punched cards into the desired categories, counting, and the tabulation or printing on appropriate forms of the classified information, can all be done mechanically. For this purpose, cards are passed through an electric sorting machine which distributes the cards in respect of any particular item of information, and at the same time counts the total number of cards falling in each group. Any number of sub-classifications can be tabulated in a very short time, and a thorough analysis of the available data made possible. The machines are also available for purposes of tabulation and printing for permanent record.

If the use of electric equipment for punching, sorting and tabulation is contemplated then much time is saved if the original information is collected in the field on carefully designed blank forms, so that the subsequent punching of information becomes almost a mechanical process. This point is important and should be carefully noted by those who have to carry out large-scale field surveys.

Experience has shown that although in a large number of cases the need for mechanical tabulation was not fully appreciated in the initial stages, it was subsequently found imperative for a satisfactory classification and tabulation of the whole mass of accumulated data. This entailed the additional labour of editing the information, i.e. copying from the original registers in a form suitable for punching thus resulting in unnecessary inconvenience, together with waste of time and money.

Hence, it is necessary to re-emphasize that irrespective of whether or not the use of mechanical sorting is contemplated, the collection of original data should be carried out on carefully designed schedules or cards. This will not only save much unnecessary writing by the field staff but, if it becomes desirable afterwards to resort to mechanical tabulation, it will make the task of subsequent analysis very much quicker, easier, and economical.

Full details of the uses of various punched cards and mechanical sorting and tabulating equipment are explained by Casey & Perry (1951).

2.4 Tabulation

The setting-out of numerical information in tabular form is a means of bringing together and presenting related material in appropriate columns or rows. A good table should not only throw into relief the important features of the data, but should also economize space and afford means by which various combinations or relationships may be easily read, compared and interpreted. Good tabulation is an art, and a careful study of the tables which appear in official publications of governments or international organizations (United Nations, 1952; World Health Organization, 1953) would help in acquiring this technique.

Tables may be drawn up purely for descriptive purposes, for comparisons, or for studying trends or changes occurring from time to time. Tables should be set out in as simple a form as possible, but should be self-explanatory and complete, i.e. not requiring reference to the text. Bigger tables should be broken up into several sections or smaller tables, rather than burdening them with too many sub-headings. The source of information should be stated either in the heading of the table or in a footnote. Explanatory notes and definitions should accompany the tables when necessary. Clarity can be introduced in tables by means of light and heavy lines, and by the use of various types and sizes of letters. In those cases in which the reliability of the basic data is limited or questionable, unnecessary digits or rates expressed in terms of a larger number of decimals tend to create an erroneous impression of high precision. For this reason only the digits which are meaningful should be retained. Tables should be numbered properly and must have suitable self-contained headings.

2.5   Frequency Distribution

After the original data have been classified according to a suitable scheme, the results are often set out in tabular form called "frequency distribution". The two columns of such a table give respectively the groups or class intervals in which the observations are classified and the number of individuals falling in each class.   It describes not only how the measurements are spread along the scale but also serves as the basis for carrying out subsequent statistical analysis.

The number of individual observations belonging to each category or class interval is called its "class frequency".   A "frequency distribution" shows the frequency with which individuals with some definite characteristic or characteristics belong to each class.   Presented in tabular form it shows the manner in which the total number of observations or the "total frequency" is distributed into various "class frequencies".   For example, measurements of wing lengths of 93 Anopheles culicifacies are shown grouped into 0.1 millimetre class intervals in the frequency distribution below (Rajindar Pal, 1945:   detailed data are quoted by Dakshinamurty, 1948).

Table 1.   Frequency distribution of wing lengths of 93 Anopheles culicifacies

Wing length (mm)	Frequency
2.05-2.14	1
2.15-2.24	1
2.25-2.34	9
2.35-2.44	14
2.45-2.54	14
2.55-2.64	20
2.65-2.74	8
2.75-2.84	18
2.85-2.94	4
2.95-3.04	2
3.05-3.14	1
3.15-3.24	0
3.25-3.34	1
Total	93

2.6   Graphic Presentation

Suitably drawn charts and diagrams provide an effective means of interpreting and presenting the results of malaria projects.   This form of presentation also helps to clarify a complex problem or reveal unnoticed relationships not otherwise obvious from the original data.   Graphs are sometimes also a means of detecting errors and omissions that may have been overlooked in a series of data.   But the use of the diagrams should not be over-emphasized.   In the words of the famous statistician Sir R. A. Fisher (1950), "Diagrams prove nothing, but bring outstanding features readily to the eye;   they are, therefore, no substitute for such critical tests as may be applied to the data, but are valuable in suggesting such tests, and in explaining the conclusions founded upon them."

Several different forms of diagrammatic presentation are available, but as far as possible in the reports of malaria survey use should be made of only the simple forms.

Although, for the preparation of diagrams, a simple set of drawing instruments is desirable, many of the diagrams explained in these notes can be easily prepared on a typewriter.

A brief description of the simple forms of diagrams is given below.

The line chart

The line chart is the one most commonly used for studying variation in malariometric indices in respect of season, years, or age.   In a line chart, time as measured in weeks, months, years, etc. is shown along the horizontal axis, called the abscissa.   The values of the quantity or indices under study are plotted, corresponding to the position on the abscissa, along the vertical axis, called the ordinate, the height of the point from the base line of the graph indicating its value.   Plotted points are connected by a solid or symbol line.   A simple example of this chart is the following (Fig. 3), in which the annual malaria morbidity rate per 1000 population (see section 3.3.3) for Ceylon has been plotted for the years 1936 to 1955.   Actual figures are given in Table 2.

Fig. 3.   Ceylon.   Annual malaria morbidity rate per 1000 population,
1936-1955

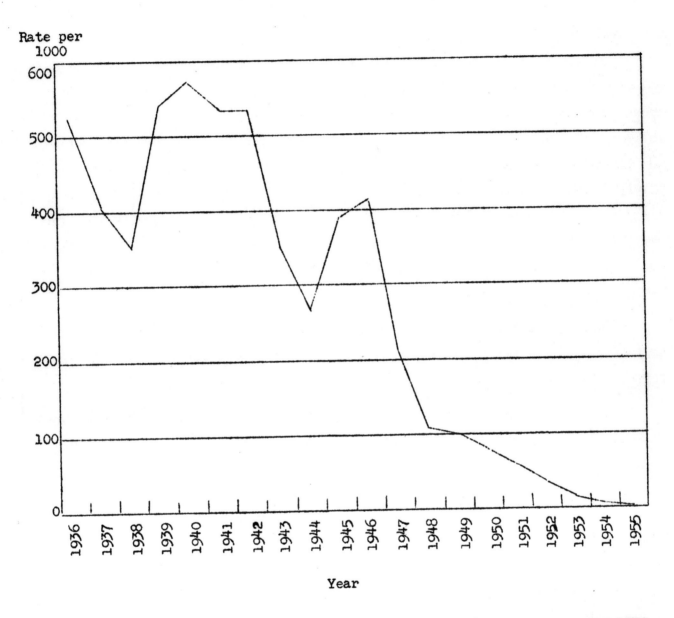

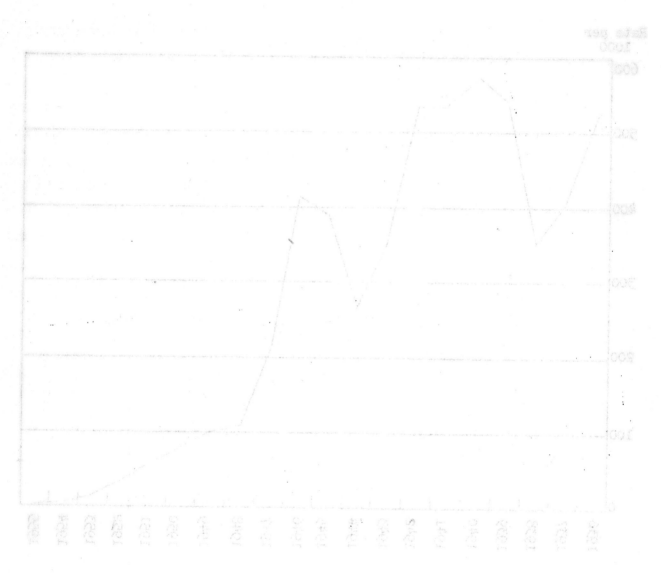

rt is recommended when emphasis is to be placed on the
ring from time to time, and particularly when several
the same chart by means of separate symbol lines.
s that if the scales along both the axes are not
can give an erroneous impression of either a very
ange.   In Figs. 4 and 5 which are examples of badly
a as given in Table 2, one of the scales chosen is much
the result that in Fig. 4 we get an impression of a
dity rate, while Fig. 5 suggests a slow decrease.
phs, therefore, the magnitude of the changes should be
nslating the points into actual figures.

. Annual malaria morbidity and mortality
1936-1955*

Year	Morbidity rate per 1000 population	Mortality rate per 100 000 population
1936	523	135
1937	404	77
1938	353	82
1939	544	170
1940	574	153
1941	535	118
1942	536	85
1943	349	110
1944	266	89
1945	391	131
1946	413	187
1947	212	66
1948	109	47
1949	100	33
1950	81	25
1951	58	21
1952	34	13
1953	11	9
1954	4	5
1955	1	5

* Source: Gunaratna (1956)

Another common mistake which leads to erroneous interpretation of line charts
is that the vertical scale may not start at zero, but at some point above it.
Fig. 6 for example, shows the trend of infant mortality rate in Chile from 1932 to
1953 (Table 3) when the ordinate starts from zero at the base line which, of course,
is the correct procedure.   If, on the other hand, the ordinate wrongly begins from
100, as in Fig. 7, the chart gives an erroneous impression of a more rapid decrease
in the rate.   Sometimes a cut may be made on the vertical axis to save space and
at the same time to warn the reader of the fact that the axis has been shortened
(see Fig. 8).

Table 3.   Chile.   Infant deaths per 1000 live births, 1932-1953

Year	Infant mortality rate
1932	235.0
1933	257.9
1934	261.9
1935	250.9
1936	252.2
1937	240.7
1938	235.7
1939	224.6
1940	217.2
1941	200.2
1942	194.7
1943	194.0
1944	180.8
1945	184.1
1946	159.5
1947	160.9
1948	160.4
1949	169.0
1950	153.0
1951	148.5
1952	133.6
1953	114.3

Fig. 4.   Ceylon.   Annual malaria morbidity rate per 1000 population
1936-1955 (abscissa contracted)

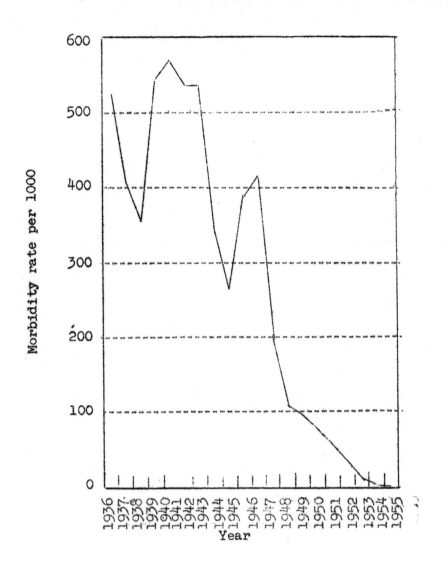

Fig. 5.   Ceylon.   Annual malaria morbidity rate per 1000 population
1936-1955 (ordinate contracted)

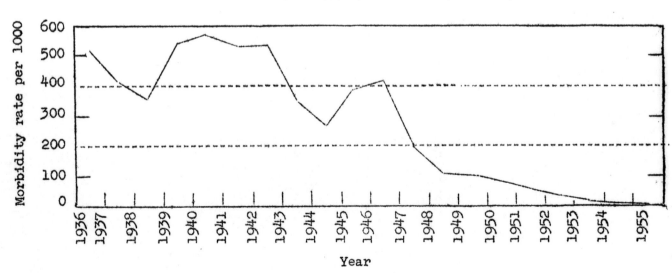

Year

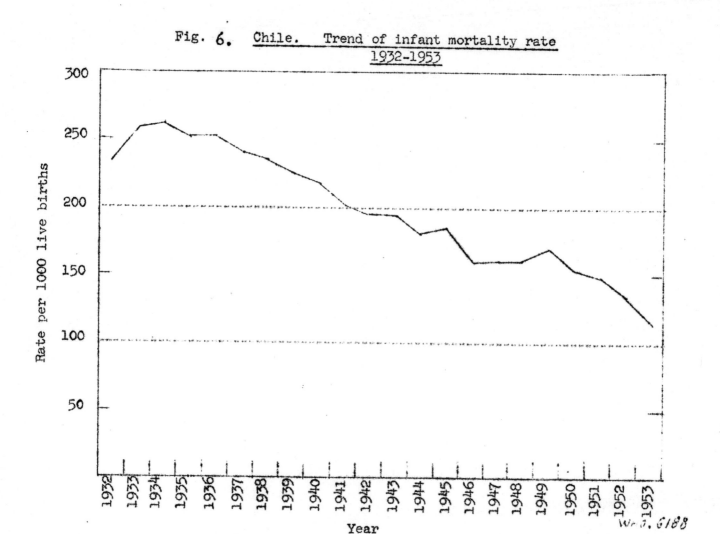

Fig. 6.   Chile.   Trend of infant mortality rate
1932-1953

Rate per 1000 live births

Year

WHO. 6188

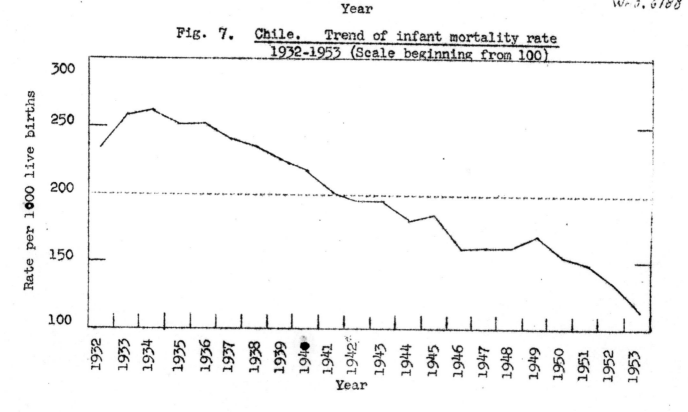

Fig. 7.   Chile.   Trend of infant mortality rate
1932-1953 (Scale beginning from 100)

Rate per 1000 live births

Year

WHO. 6189

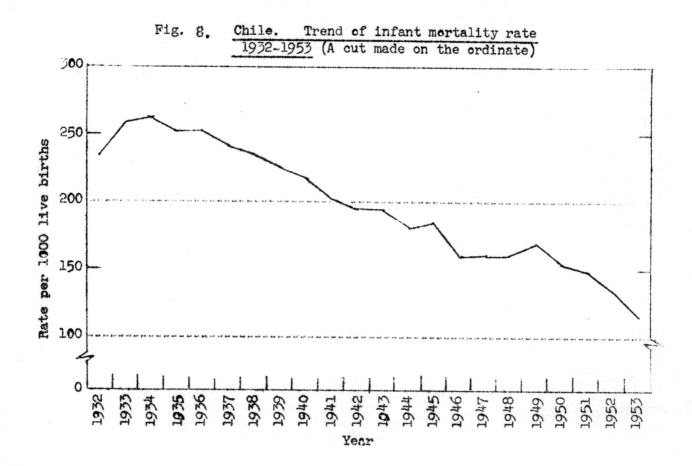

Fig. 8.   Chile.   Trend of infant mortality rate
1932-1953 (A cut made on the ordinate)

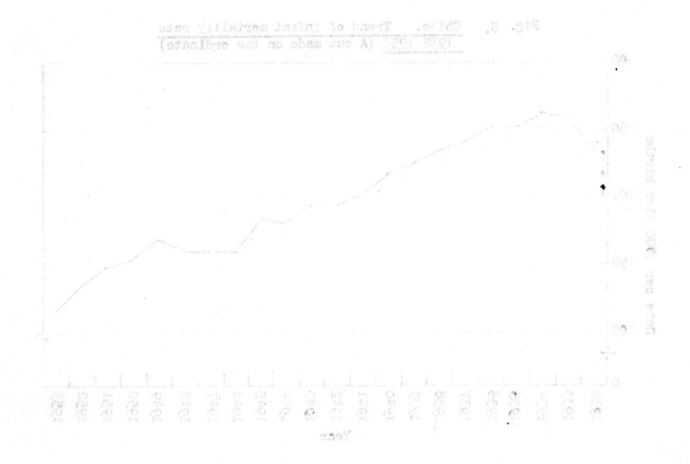

Fig. 8.   Chile.   Trend of infant mortality rate
1929-1951 (A cut made on the ordinate)

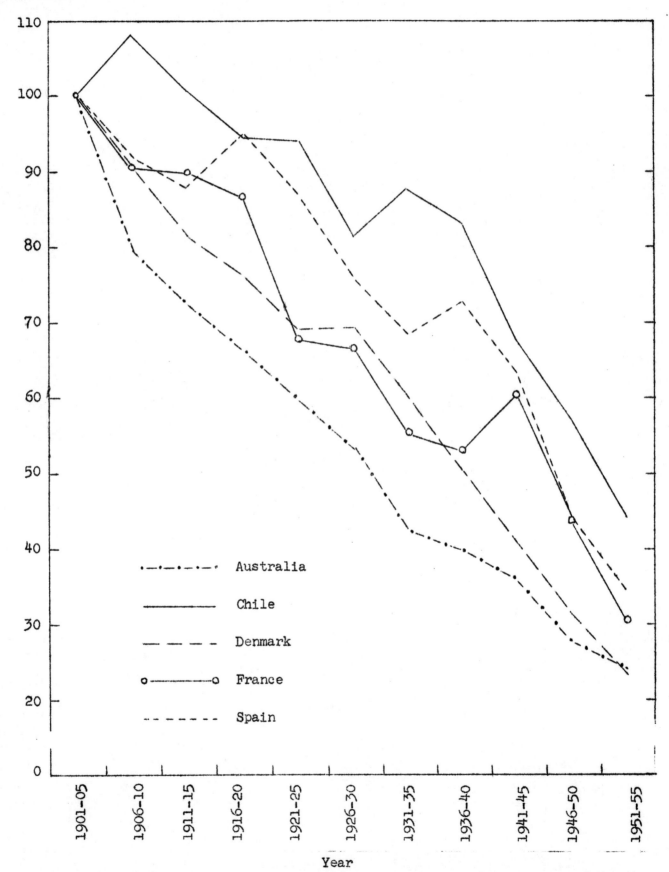

Fig. 9. Trend of five-year-average infant mortality rate
in certain countries, 1901-1955
(Average rate for 1901-05 taken as 100)

Percentage

110

100

90

80

70

60

50

40

30

20

0

1901-05 1906-10 1911-15 1916-20 1921-25 1926-30 1931-35 1936-40 1941-45 1946-50 1951-55

Year

- — · — · — · Australia

——————— Chile

— — — — Denmark

o —— o France

- - - - - Spain

WHO 7331

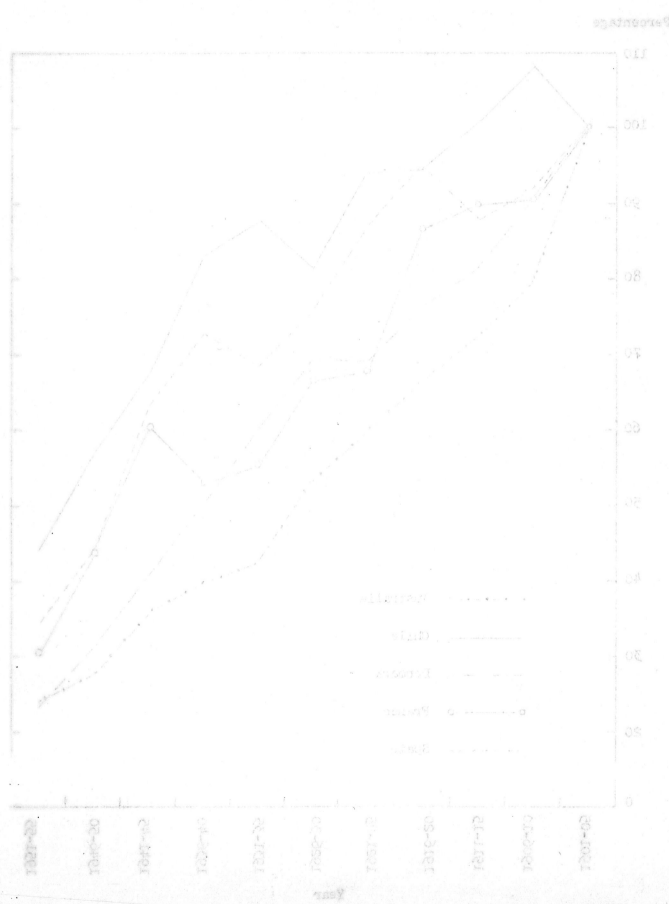

Fig. 10. Ceylon. Trend of crude death rate and malaria death rate
1936-1955

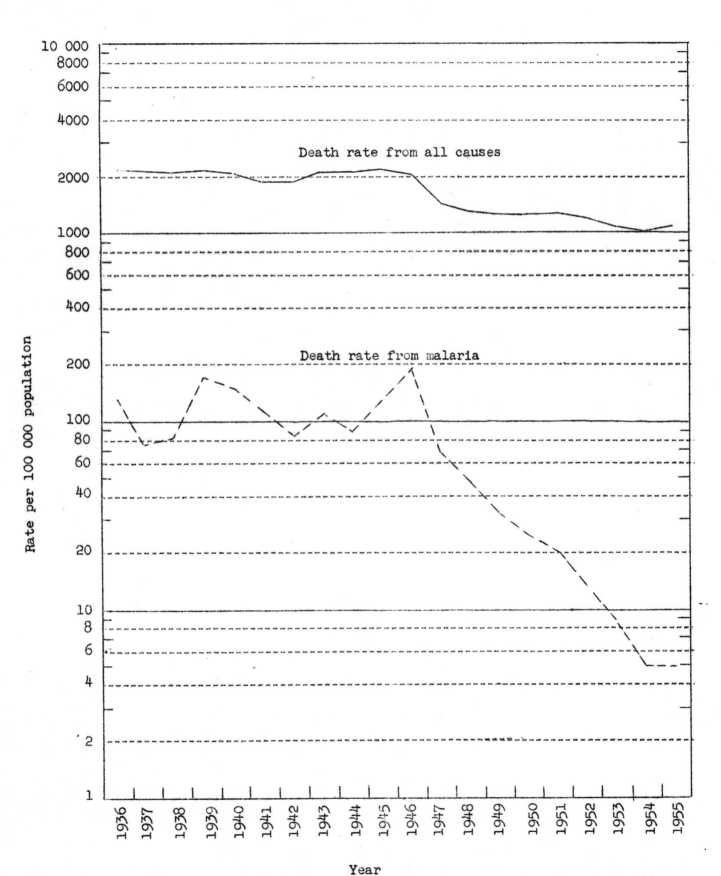

Death rate from all causes

Death rate from malaria

Rate per 100 000 population

Year

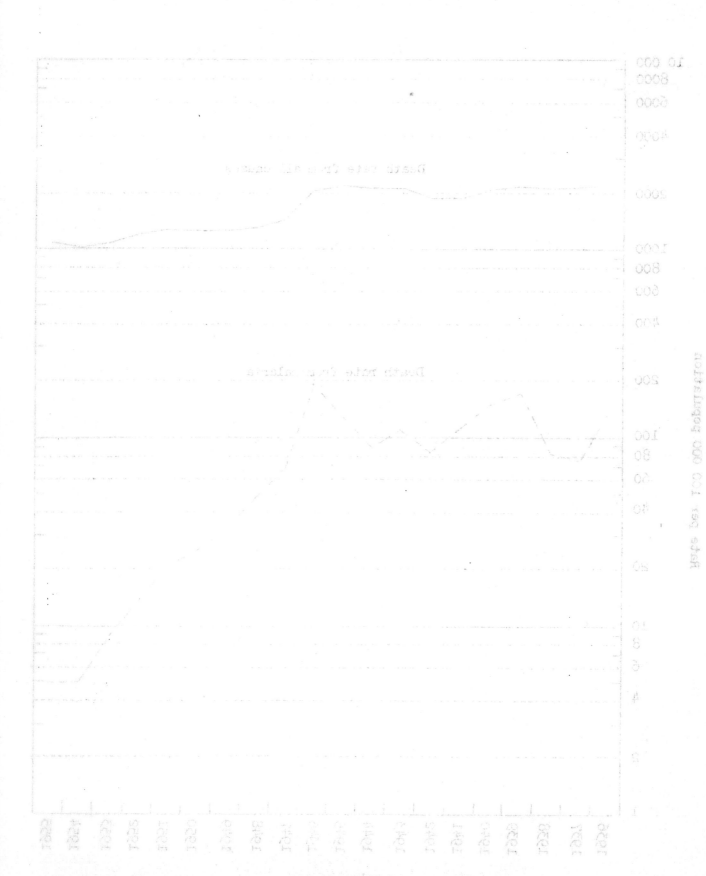

Fig. 10.   Ceylon. Trend ? crude death rate and malaria death rate
1920-1955

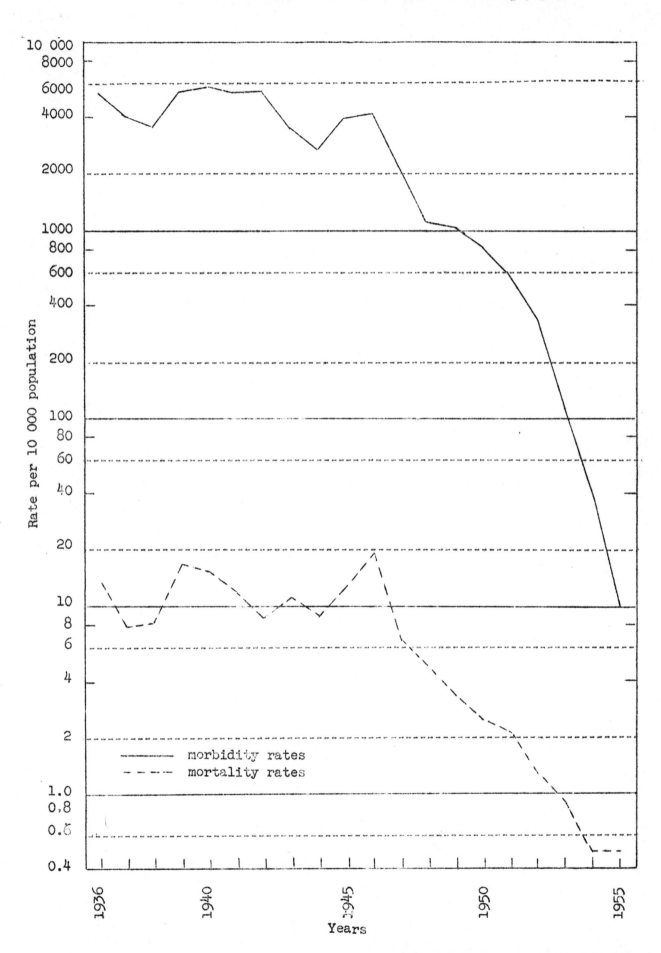

Fig. 11. Ceylon. Annual malaria morbidity and malaria mortality rates per 10 000, 1936-1955, on semilog paper

WHO 7326

Another use of the line chart is in connexion with the study of indices beginning with a common base. For instance, in Fig. 9 the trend of five-year average infant mortality rate (section 3.3.3) in certain countries from 1901 to 1955 has been plotted by converting all rates as percentages of the average rate for 1901-1905. The purpose of plotting such indices is to place all countries which were at differing levels of infant mortality rate in 1901-1905 on a common base. Such charts are useful for comparing the trend of indices relative to some basic year between two or more series which may differ considerably in amount or quantity, or when the relationship of two or more series of unlike basic units is to be shown.

In connexion with the use of scales, a device sometimes found useful is to mark the ordinate with the logarithmic scale, as is shown in Fig. 10. The purpose of this chart is not to show the actual amount of change, but to study the rate of change between two consecutive periods in a series of figures. The slope of lines connecting the plotted points on a semilog chart indicates the rate of change, i.e. the steeper the rise or fall of these lines, the greater is the ratio of increase or decrease from one point to the next. For instance, we may plot annual figures of malaria death rate and crude death rate (i.e. death rate from all causes) by two lines on the same chart. The question to be studied is whether annual change in both the total death rate and the malaria death rate is similar, or whether there has been some tendency for the two to vary differently as would happen for instance if the malaria deaths decreased faster owing to an extensive campaign. When both the crude death rate and the malaria death rate are shown on a logarithmic scale their relative variation becomes readily apparent to the eye. Charts of this type are usually called semilog charts, because only one of the scales shows logarithmic figures. Another example of the use of semilogarithmic charts would be to examine whether in a given population malaria cases and malaria deaths have both decreased at the same relative rate or not. This is shown for Ceylon in Fig. 11. From 1946 onwards the decrease in malaria morbidity has been relatively more rapid.

An interesting example of logarithmic scale for studying reduction in malaria morbidity from year to year is provided by Boyd (1949) page 864.

It is to be noted that on the semilogarithmic paper the ordinate scale does not begin with zero but with unity.   In other words, zero figures cannot be shown on this scale.   Likewise, negative values cannot be plotted on a logarithmic scale.

Semilogarithmic printed sheets are usually obtainable from local draughting or stationery supply stores.

The bar diagram

The underlying principle in the construction of a bar diagram is that magnitudes to be compared are shown by proportional lengths of bars.   The bar diagram is useful for studying the relative values of individual countries or population groups, etc. as illustrated by Fig. 12 in which malaria death rates per 100 000 inhabitants are shown for 20 countries in the Americas.   The figure is reproduced from a paper by Molina & Puffer (1955).   The bars originate at the right of a common base line and are measured along the horizontal axis.   The name of the population group or category is usually stated on the left of the bar.   As far as possible it is advisable to arrange these bars in decreasing order of magnitude although sometimes it may be considered more expedient to arrange the categories in alphabetical order.   When they are shown in descending order it can clearly be seen which population groups, etc. are above or below the average or what position they occupy among all groups with regard to the magnitude of the measurement.   In an alphabetical arrangement the bars appear irregular, although each population group can be more readily located.   This form of diagrammatic representation is sometimes also used for plotting figures in respect of time when only a few selected dates or periods are to be shown.   In that case, of course, the bars should be arranged chronologically and stand vertically over a horizontal base line.   The bar diagram should not be used to depict a consecutive trend of a series over a long period of time;   the line chart being more suited for this type of data.   On the other hand, a line chart cannot be used to give values of different countries unless they are of chronological type.

Sometimes against each area more than one measurement may be shown as, for instance, would happen if we were to show malaria death rates separately for rural and urban populations or infant mortality rates separately by sex.   If the infant mortality rate were to be shown by several economic groups for each area, the number of bars

Fig. 12. <u>Deaths from malaria per 100 000 population in
20 countries of the Americas, 1952</u>

<u>Country</u>   <u>Deaths per 100 000 population</u>

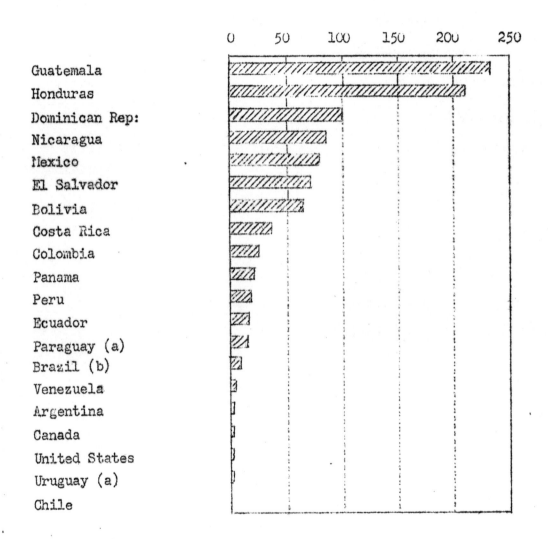

(a)   1951

(b)   Federal districts and State capitals, with
      the exception of the city of São Paulo.

Fig. 1a   Deaths from malaria per 100 000 population in
20 countries of the Americas, 1968

Country   Deaths per 100 000 population

                          50   100   150   200   250

Guatemala
Honduras
Dominican Rep.
Nicaragua
Mexico
El Salvador
Bolivia
Costa Rica
Colombia
Panama
Peru
Ecuador
Paraguay (a)
Brazil (b)
Venezuela
Argentina
Canada
United States
Uruguay (a)
Chile

(a) 1967

(b) Federal districts and states of ... 1815, with
     the exception of the city of Rio ...

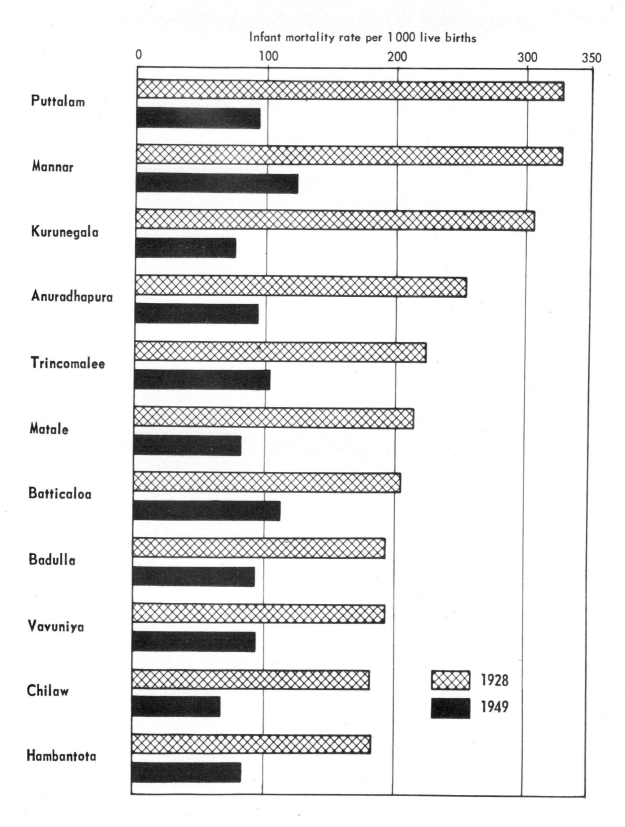

Fig. 13 Ceylon. Infant mortality rate in the years 1928 and 1949 in districts lying in the hyperendemic malaria zone

WHO 7321

corresponding to each place may be large.   As far as possible, the number of bars should be limited to three or four as more than that number tends to give a confusing picture.   A marked contrast in shading the bars for different categories should be used to distinguish them from each other.   Fig. 13 is an example of such a diagram where for each district two bars correspond to two different time periods.

The map diagram

For depicting geographical variation or distribution in space, maps are used. As an example the geographical variation of death rate from all causes during the malaria epidemic of 1934-1935 in Ceylon is shown in Fig. 14 (Ceylon, 1935). Different areas are shaded or cross-hatched, as shown in the illustration.   The shaded portion should run progressively from dark to light, depending upon the emphasis desired in the data.   By arranging the data in numerical order an indication is obtained as to which degree of shading should be allocated to the different indices. This shading pattern should be sufficiently distinctive to show clearly the differences in area.   As few patterns as possible should be used and the number may not exceed 5 or 6.   In so far as only a few categories are used for shading purposes, a good deal of information is sacrificed.   This form of diagrammatic representation should therefore be adopted only when a study of the geographical distribution is of importance.   Otherwise it is preferable to use bar diagrams.

The use of map diagrams is appropriate, strictly speaking, only when the data to be presented in a surface map are definitely in terms of the area, as for instance to show mortality or morbidity by districts, density of population, rainfall by regions, etc.

If our interest lies not in showing the absolute magnitude, but certain qualifying data as, for instance, the prevailing species of mosquitos, different types of symbols may be used to mark the places in the map.

2.6.1 Graphic presentation of frequency distributions

It is usual to show a frequency distribution by means of a diagram (called histogram) illustrated in Fig. 15, in which the horizontal axis relates to wing length in millimetres, and the height of each bar raised on the corresponding class interval is proportional to the frequency value in that class interval. More precisely, the area of each rectangle corresponds to the frequency in that particular interval. Thus, when the class intervals are of equal magnitude, as in the example discussed, the height of each bar is proportional to the corresponding class frequency. If, on the other hand, the class intervals are unequal, we have to be careful in marking the heights of the bars so as to ensure that the area of the bar raised on a class interval corresponds to the frequency of that interval. For example, in the case of any class intervals being double the others, the height of the bar will be reduced to half.

If the variable is measured along the horizontal axis, as in the case of the histogram, but the frequency for each class interval is marked by a point along the vertical axis and these points are joined by lines, then we get what is called a "frequency polygon", (see Fig. 16). The points should be plotted corresponding to the middle points of class intervals.

If the number of observations are relatively large, and if these measurements are classified in smaller class intervals, both histogram and frequency polygon tend to lose their irregularities caused by haphazard observations and tend to assume the shape of a smooth curve called a "frequency curve", (see Fig. 17).

In the example of the wing length of Anopheles culicifacies (section 2.5) the frequency curve is nearly symmetrical, but it is not infrequent to come across data which assume non-symmetric or what are called "skew" shapes.

The spread of the histogram or frequency lygon on either side of the peak indicates the degree of variability in the recorded measurements. If the majority of measurements tend to be alike, then owing to a clustering of the observation near the average value, the diagram is relatively peaked. If, on the other hand, the individual measurements exhibit a great deal of variation, the curve will tend to flatten out on either side. This point is illustrated by means of two histograms

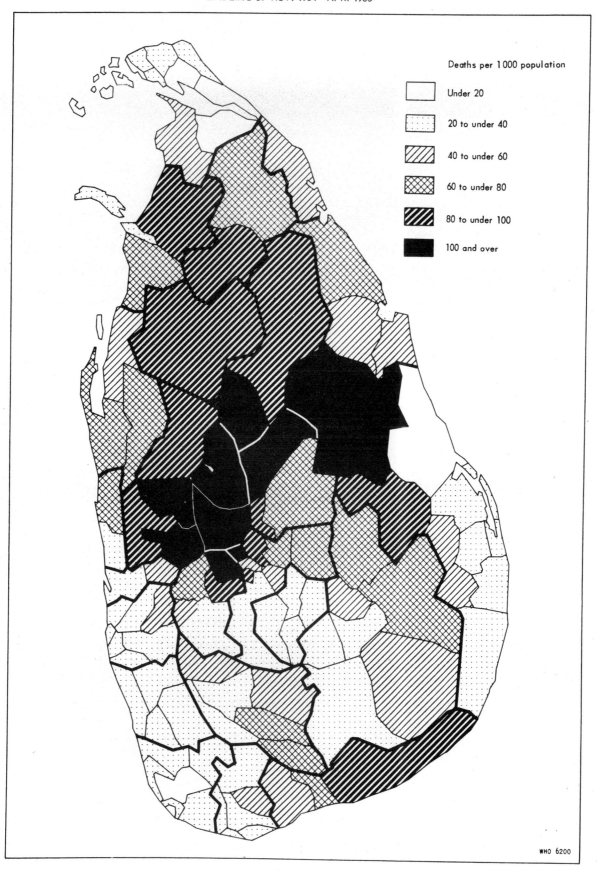

FIG. 14   CEYLON. GEOGRAPHICAL VARIATION OF DEATH RATE FROM ALL CAUSES DURING THE MALARIA
EPIDEMIC OF NOV. 1934 - APR. 1935

Deaths per 1000 population

Under 20

20 to under 40

40 to under 60

60 to under 80

80 to under 100

100 and over

WHO 6200

Fig. 15.   Histogram of wing lengths of 93 Anopheles culicifacies

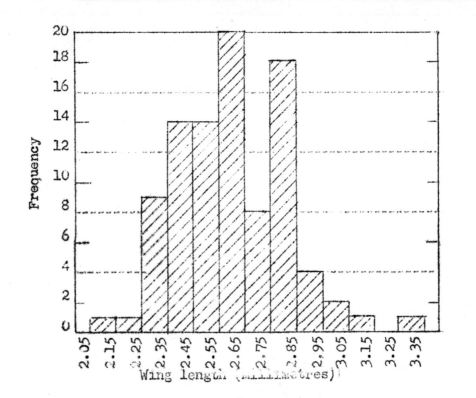

WHO.6196

Fig. 16.   Frequency polygon of wing lengths of 93
Anopheles culicifacies

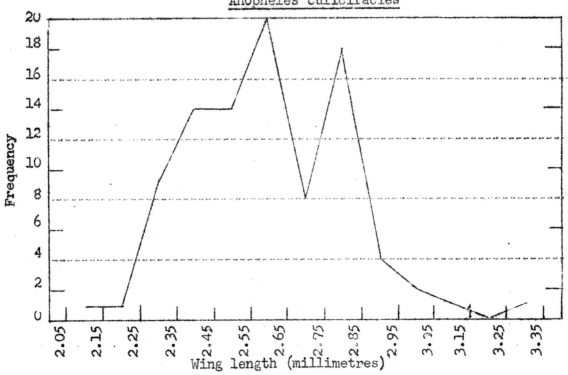

WHO.6197

Fig. 17. Normal curve fitted to the frequency distribution of wing lengths of 93 Anopheles culicifacies

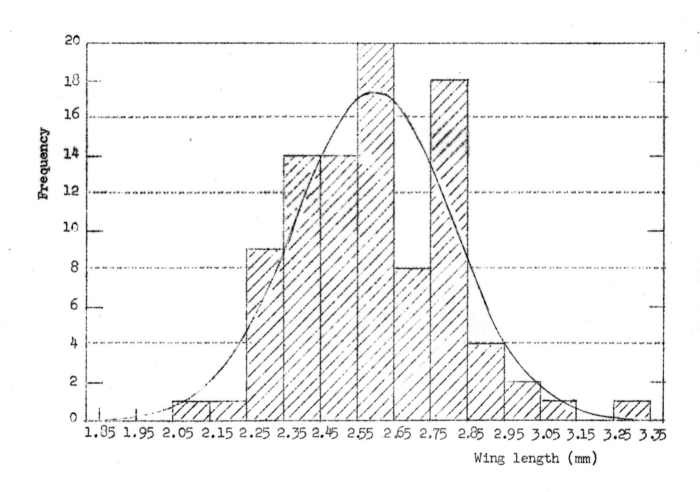

Fig. 17. Normal curve fitted to the frequency distribution of wing lengths of 97 Anopheles culicifacies

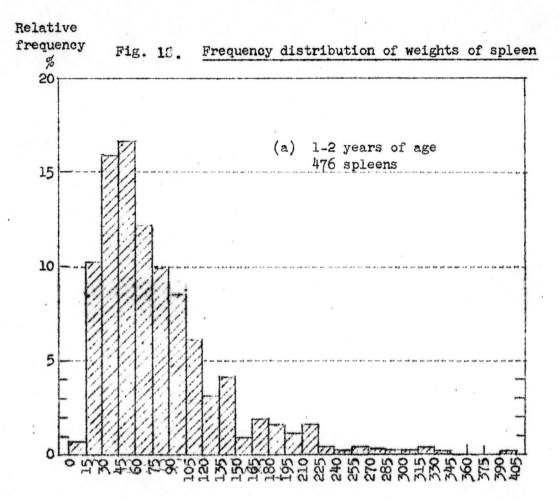

Fig. 18. Frequency distribution of weights of spleen

(a) 1-2 years of age
     476 spleens

Spleen weight (grammes)

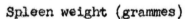
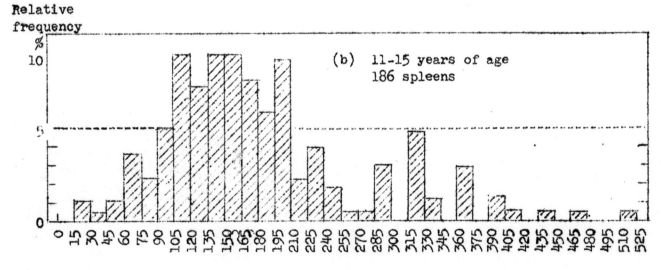

(b) 11-15 years of age
     186 spleens

Spleen weight (grammes)

WHO. 5212

Fig. 12. Frequency distribution of weights of spleen

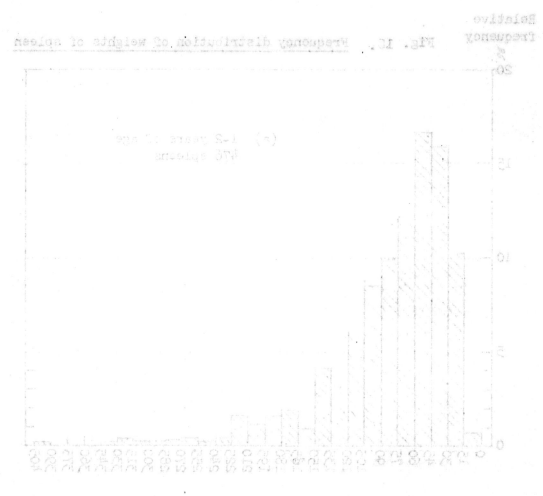

(a) 1-2 years of age
476 spleens

Spleen weight (grammes)

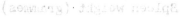

Relative
frequency
%

(b) 12-15 years of age
181 spleens

Spleen weight (grammes)

of differing peakedness in Fig. 18.   These diagrams show the weight of spleen found
on autopsies of African infants.   One relates to 476 infants of 1-2 years of age
and the other to 186 children of 11-15 years of age (Bruce-Chwatt, 1956).   Since
these two groups include different numbers of children, the diagrams are drawn to
show, instead of the frequency itself, the relative frequency, i.e. the proportion
of each class frequency to the total number of children in each group, so that the
relative magnitude of the class frequency is directly comparable between the two
groups.   It is seen that the histogram relating to the 11-15 years group is situated
more on the right side, which incidentally exhibits the fact that on the average
this group had heavier spleens.   What is of special interest is the fact that the
histogram of the 11-15 years group is relatively more spread out than the other,
indicating thereby a greater degree of variability among the spleen weights for this
age-group than the other.   This comparison stresses the point that when studying a
set of observations one should not only consider the average value but also pay
regard to the degree of variability in the whole set of observations.   It is not
unusual to come across cases where two histograms may have their peaks coinciding
and yet one may be more spread out than the other.   Indeed, statistical methods are
available by means of which the degree of spread among a set of measurements can be
numerically expressed by a single figure, which in statistical terminology is called
"variance" (the term is explained in section 2.13), so that the variability of one
or more frequency distributions can be statistically compared (see section 2.17).

2.7   Normal Curve

Among the various types of frequency curves there is one which is of considerable
importance in statistical analysis.   It is called the normal curve.   This curve is
symmetrical in shape, resembling that shown in the diagram relating to the distribution
of wing lengths of 93 Anopheles culicifacies (Fig. 17).   The shape of the normal
curve is mathematically defined by the following formula:

$$f(x) = \frac{1}{\sqrt{2\pi}\,\sigma} \; e^{-\frac{1}{2\sigma^2}(x-m)^2}$$

where   x : value of variable

     f(x) : height of the frequency curve at x

      π = 3.14159 ...

      e = 2.71828 ...

      m, σ are constants, viz. the mean and the standard deviation
              (explained later in sections 2.12 and 2.13)

To illustrate its shape, a normal curve is shown in Fig. 17 superposed on the histogram of 93 wing lengths. In order to fit this curve to the recorded data, the statistician proceeds by estimating the values of m and σ from the original observations. The technique of fitting the curve is beyond the scope of these notes. The method is explained in paragraph 8.7 of Snedecor (1956).

It is indeed of considerable interest to study the frequency distribution and the corresponding frequency curve of measurements collected in connexion with malaria work. This point is well emphasized in the following quotation from "Malaria Terminology", (Covell et al., 1953) page 39:

"Data giving the number of enlarged spleens of different measurements can be studied from the point of view of frequency distribution of the classes. Such frequency distribution, unlike the parasite infection frequency, is well displayed in frequency curves of the usual type. The curve given is a valuable aid to the study of splenomegaly in malaria, since the frequency distribution of different classes of spleen is the fundamental phenomenon on which such values as the average enlarged spleen are dependent."

2.8   Statistical Techniques for analysing Data

Data collected by malaria workers may be classified broadly into two types:

(i)   qualitative data, as for instance, the number of persons attacked and not attacked with malaria, the number of children with or without splenic enlargement, etc. and specifically such entomological observations as development of ovarian follicles or the appearance of wing fringes for both of which certain categories have been suggested by Covell et al. (1953): such data permit of the classification of individuals belonging to one of several different categories specified qualitatively;

(ii)   quantitative observations or measurements such as the size of the spleen measured in centimetres, ages of children, parasite counts, etc., measures which are expressed in numerical terms.

Statistical techniques of a simple kind for dealing with these two types of data are discussed separately in the pages that follow.   The discussion presented here is brief, the purpose being firstly to indicate the broad lines on which the analysis may be begun, and secondly to introduce and explain statistical terminology commonly encountered in scientific and malariometric literature.   Further exposition of these elementary methods will be found in the book: "Principles of Medical Statistics" by A. Bradford Hill (1955).

Although the techniques described are of fairly general applicability, it must be pointed out that each has its own limitations.   For instance, many methods presume that the data are of such a kind as would be distributed according to the normal frequency curve.   In other words, some of these techniques may be inapplicable if the observed frequency distribution is of an asymmetrical type.   Certain tests presume that the number of observations is fairly large.   Almost invariably, the very important assumption is made that when a sample of children are examined, or blood cells or any other individual units are measured, the individual measurements are independent of each other.

2.9   Qualitative Data

The simplest example of qualitative classification is that obtained when a group of individuals is classed in two categories as, for example, children with or without enlarged spleen, female anopheles showing or not showing sporozoites on dissection of the salivary glands, malaria patients treated or untreated, patients relieved of clinical symptoms or died, etc.   In such cases our interest generally lies in comparing the proportion of the total showing certain characteristics with a similar proportion calculated under a different situation.   As an example we may be interested in comparing the percentages of children with enlarged spleen for two areas, for two different age-groups, for the two sexes, or at two different times.

Such data relating to two population groups and again classified for each group into
two categories are usually tabulated in the following form of what is called a
"2 x 2" table, or a "four-fold" table in which the four cells of the table relate to
mutually exclusive categories.   This tabular presentation is also called "double-
dichotomous".   As a specific example let us consider the following data (Table 4)
obtained on spleen examination of male and female children (age 2-9 years) for an
area.

Table 4.   Children with and without spleen enlargement
by sex (aged 2-9 years)

	Children with enlarged spleen	Children without enlarged spleen	Total	Spleen rate
Male	21	59	80	26%
Female	37	63	100	37%
Total	58	122	180	32%

From this table it is apparent that female children had a higher spleen rate in so
far as those 180 children under observation are concerned.   But generally we are not
merely concerned with knowing the spleen rate for just these 180 children.   The real
aim of such a survey is to compare the spleen rates for the entire child population
in the area, on the presumption that the observations made on the 180 children provided
an adequate and representative sample of the whole child population.   In other words,
presuming that the sample was representative, we should ask ourselves to what extent
the results of examinations on a sample of the population can be generalized.

Estimates of the spleen rate shown in this example for the two sexes are based
on small numbers, viz. 80 and 100 children.   If the selection of the sample was biased,
for instance if only the children attending school were examined to the exclusion of
those confined to bed because of malaria, such findings would obviously be unsuitable
for any generalization for the area.   Even when the sample involves no known or
unknown bias, it is not unlikely that another group of children examined from the

same age-group may give somewhat different rates for the two sexes, which again may differ from the rates obtained on examining all the children. Thus some variation in the two rates is expected to arise from the fact that we have not examined all the children but only a sample of them. The question we ask is, are the spleen rates of the two sexes really different, recognizing that both these rates are liable to some variation from errors of sampling?

It may be observed that a similar problem of comparing two percentages can arise in a large variety of studies whether they relate to schoolchildren, mosquito population, cases treated in a hospital, etc. The general technique for dealing with such situations is explained with respect to the example given above. In order to examine whether the two percentages are really different, we begin by making the hypothesis that the two rates are not essentially different. This is the conventional method by which the statistician would invariably begin his analysis. He then examines the observed results to see if, on the basis of the accepted theory of probability, the difference could be due to chance variation. If he finds that there is very little possibility that the difference could be due to chance, the hypothesis that the rates are not different is disproved. Similarly, when two treatments have been tried on two similar groups of patients and the numbers of patients who recovered and did not recover have been recorded in the 2 x 2 table, the statistician begins by postulating the hypothesis that the two treatments were alike in their effects and he proceeds to examine this hypothesis according to the probability theory to see if the observed results can at all contradict it. Such a hypothesis is called the "null hypothesis". Only if a further statistical scrutiny of the data can contradict the "null hypothesis" can the difference in the two groups be considered real, that is, the possibility that chance alone could have produced the difference in the two groups is then ruled out. If, on the other hand, it can be shown that the results obtained were such as could be observed from chance alone fairly frequently on the basis of the null hypothesis, then the observed difference in the two groups, however large, will not be regarded as a genuine difference. Statistical theory shows that if a difference really exists the relative importance of chance factors in causing such a difference diminishes as the size of the sample becomes greater.

It should therefore be clearly understood that if owing to the smallness of the
sample size the data fail to contradict the null hypothesis of the statistician,
the experimental evidence should be regarded as inadequate from the statistical
point of view.   Indeed, before any investigation is undertaken, a knowledge of
the null hypothesis which the statistician will postulate and which he will expect
the experimental data to contradict categorically, should provide a helpful guide
to workers in the proper planning of their experiments.   Of course, the manner in
which a contradiction of the null hypothesis will be sought by the statistician
should also be known to experimental workers before they embark upon the actual
conduct of the experiments or survey.

2.10   Statistical Significance

The method of reasoning adopted in all statistical tests of significance is
similar and is well illustrated by the analysis carried out on the figures of a
four-fold table.   Generally, our aim is to discriminate between one or more
alternate hypotheses regarding the factors which might have produced the observed
difference in results.   For instance, the differences may be either due to the
factor under study (sex differences, treatment differences, place differences, etc.),
or to some very important and perhaps unknown factor such as a strong bias in the
selection of the subjects under study, or due to the play of a number of small
uncontrolled and uncontrollable circumstances such as those which cannot be overcome in experiments on living subjects.   Generally, the last set of factors are
discriminated by the term "randomness" or "chance" or sampling errors.   It is
believed that in the event of the two groups being otherwise similar, i.e. the null
hypothesis being true, and with only random factors being at play, some variation
in the observed results of the two groups will be expected.   We therefore proceed
to assess the probability of randomness alone having produced the observed difference.
In so doing we ask ourselves the question that if the same experiment or survey were
to be repeated theoretically an infinitely large number of times under similar
conditions, with both groups otherwise kept under identical conditions, on how many
occasions would we observe differences as large as, or even larger than those
actually observed?   At first thought it might seem that for this purpose the
experiment or the survey will have to be repeated an infinitely large number of times -

an obvious impracticability.   This, however, is not necessary.   The answer is
provided by the mathematical theory of probability.   From this theory we can know
in what proportion of cases randomness alone will produce results as divergent or
even more divergent than those observed.   If, on the basis of this theory we find
that the observed differences can occur from chance in only as few cases as five
out of 100 (.05 chance), we can safely assert that in the case actually observed
the difference is not a chance occurrence.   Some workers may be more stringent in
their demand, and stipulate that only if such a divergent result, or an even more
divergent result can arise from chance only in as low as 1 per cent. cases (.01 chance),
would we be justified in excluding randomness as the possible cause of having brought
about the observed difference.   Of course, we have no method of judging whether the
observed result is one of these five rare occasions (or in the more stringent case,
1 in 100 occasions) on which chance alone would produce the observed result, but since
the ratio of 5:95 (or 1:99) is relatively very small, we presume that there is greater
justification for ascribing the observed difference in the result to some other cause,
and for recording the null hypothesis as contradicted.

It must be pointed out that even if the statistical significance of the observed
difference is thus established, it does not necessarily carry with it the implication
that the differential effect was brought about definitely and only by the factor under
study.   Thus, if the difference in the spleen rate was proved to be statistically
significant between male and female children, statistical examination can only
indicate whether or not chance could have accounted for the observed difference.
Once this possibility of chance is allowed for, it remains for the experimental
worker to examine whether the observed difference is to be ascribed to the factor he
has studied, i.e. the sex difference only, or possibly to some other cause.   He must
examine whether male and female children were similar in ages, socio-economic status,
etc.   If both groups were examined for spleen enlargement separately at different
periods, the time factor itself may have brought about the difference.   If male
children were generally examined in the school and female children at home, or the
male children happened to be examined in the recumbent position and the female
children in an erect posture, other factors of selection would affect the findings.

Thus, without an intimate knowledge of the causes that can affect the results, a satisfactory judgement on the cause of the difference cannot always be given. Factors such as age, weight, sex, presence of disease in one group, and in many cases a bias from unknown causes affecting the initial selection of the two groups differently may sometimes introduce considerable differences. Before undertaking any survey it is therefore essential that the effect of such factors as are likely to influence the results should be carefully foreseen and as far as possible eliminated. The one satisfactory method of ensuring absence of bias is to select the groups strictly by a procedure which in statistical terminology is called "random". For this purpose a complete list of the children in the area is first prepared separately for the two sexes. Then each child is given a serial number in the list. Each number may then be written on a small card and the whole pack thoroughly mixed or shuffled. Then similar to the process of drawing a lottery, we draw as many cards as the number of children to be included in the sample. The serial numbers appearing in the selected group are then of those children who should be examined. In Appendix B are provided numbers arranged in a random order, which can be utilized for random sampling. The use of these numbers is explained also in section 2.20.1.

As is explained in section 5, the precision of the results is improved by increasing the number of children to be examined. It is necessary to include an adequate number of children in the study which in some cases may mean the examination of all the children of the village, or of two or more epidemiologically similar neighbouring villages.

2.11 Chi-square (X^2) Test

In the present example (Table 4), on the basis of our null hypothesis we first regard the two groups as similar, and therefore estimate a single spleen rate for the total number of 180 male and female children. Since there were 58 children with enlarged spleen, the combined spleen rate is:

$$\frac{58}{180} \times 100 = 32.22\%$$

In fact, on the basis of available data this is the best estimate we can make of the spleen rate for the entire group. If this rate was true for both male and female children we should have expected that out of 80 male children $\frac{32.22 \times 80}{100} = 25.78$ or about 26 children would have shown enlarged spleen. Following the same argument, we should have expected $\frac{(32.22 \times 100)}{100} = 32.22$ or about 32 female children to have shown enlargement of spleen instead of the 37 actually observed. Are these differences between the expected numbers (called E) and those actually observed (called O) in the four cells of any statistical significance? To answer this question we proceed to calculate what is called the "chi-square" (χ^2). The values of observed numbers of children with or without spleen enlargement and those expected on the basis of the null hypothesis are shown below separately for each cell.

With enlargement of the spleen		Without enlargement of the spleen	
Male	Observed O = 21	Observed = 59	
	Expected E = 25.78	Expected = 54.22	
	O - E = -4.78	O - E = +4.78	
	$(O - E)^2/E = 0.886$	$(O - E)^2/E = 0.421$	
Female	Observed = 37	Observed = 63	
	Expected = 32.22	Expected = 67.78	
	O - E = +4.78	O - E = -4.78	
	$(O - E)^2/E = 0.709$	$(O - E)^2/E = 0.337$	

$$\chi^2 = 0.886 + 0.421 + 0.709 + 0.337$$
$$= 2.353$$

Each difference between the observed and expected value is squared and divided by the expected value as has been done above for each of the four cells separately.

The value of chi-square is then obtained by adding these values.

$$\chi^2 = \Sigma \frac{(0 - E)^2}{E}$$

where Σ (the Greek capital letter sigma) indicates that the values obtained for all the four cells are added.

It will be clear that if the divergence between the observed and expected values is of a very low order the quantity $(0 - E)^2$ or $\frac{(0 - E)^2}{E}$ will all be very small. Of course, if the observed values were exactly the same as expected from our null hypothesis then $0 - E$ will be zero as also will be the value of chi-square. On the other hand, if the observed values depart considerably from those expected on the basis of our null hypothesis the difference $(0 - E)$ will be large in each cell, thus contributing to a high value of chi-square. In chi-square, therefore, we have a single numerical measure of the departure of observed series from the expected value under our null hypothesis. The larger the value of chi-square the more justification will there be for us to think that our null hypothesis is not supported by the observations because they departed too far from it.

The value of chi-square is judged in relation to a probability scale where we try to think of the chances of the null hypothesis being contradicted by the data. A very large value of chi-square shows that the probability of our results being consistent with the null hypothesis is practically zero, which means that we were not justified in assuming that the two groups were similar. If for a 2 x 2 table the chi-square were as high as 10.827 (a figure derived from probability theory), then it is known from probability theory that there is only one chance in a thousand that such a divergence as is noted in the 2 x 2 table or even greater divergence if possible will be obtained on the basis of our null hypothesis. This indeed is a low probability. In that case we will be justified in concluding that the two groups were different. If the value of chi-square was as high as 6.635, then we know from probability theory that the chance of our observations being consistent with the null hypothesis is only 1 in 100, again a low probability value. If the value of chi-square obtained from a 2 x 2 table were 3.841 then there would be only 5 per cent. chance of our data being consistent with the null hypothesis. A chi-square equal to 2.706 corresponds on the probability scale to 10 per cent. chance only of the observations being consistent with the null hypothesis. It is a convention among statisticians that if the value of chi-square equals or exceeds that corresponding to 5 per cent. probability level, i.e. if it is 3.841 or more, we consider that the null hypothesis is contradicted. Some experimental workers prefer to lay a more stringent test by accepting the 1 per cent. probability level which implies that the chi-square should be 6.635 or more in order to reject the null hypothesis. If therefore the value of chi-square found from a four-fold table is smaller than 3.841 (5 per cent. level of significance) as is the case in the above example, the statistician argues that the observed data could reasonably have also arisen from chance even if there were no real difference, i.e. the data failed to contradict his null hypothesis. In that case the justification is not strong enough for regarding the two groups as statistically different from each other.

The computational work involved in finding out the value of chi-square from a 2 x 2 table is considerably shortened and the need for working out expected values for individual cells and squaring the differences, etc. completely obviated by adopting the following formula which yields a value identical to that of chi-square obtained by the method described above.

$$\chi^2 = \frac{(ad - bc)^2 (N)}{(a + b)(c + d)(a + c)(b + d)},$$

where a, b, c and d are numbers belonging to the four cells of the 2 x 2 table as shown below:

a c	a + c
b d	b + d
a+b c+d	a+b+c+d = N

The corresponding figures from Table 4 are as follows:

21 59	80
37 63	100
58 122	180

With this numerical example we proceed as follows:

Step 1.   Find the difference between the cross-product of the cell values (ad - bc).
In the example above the two cross-products of the cell values are 21 x 63 and
59 x 37.   Their difference is 21 x 63 - 59 x 37 = 1323 - 2183 = -860.

Step 2.   Square the differences obtained in step 1 and multiply by the total number
of observations $(ad - bc)^2 N = (-860)^2 \times 180 = 133\ 128\ 000$.

Step 3.   Divide the quantity obtained in step 2 by the product of the four marginal
totals:

$$\frac{133\ 128\ 000}{80 \times 100 \times 122 \times 58} = 2.352$$

which is the value of chi-square and agrees well with the value 2.353 obtained by
the more laborious computation described earlier.   (The difference of 0.001 has
arisen from the rounding off of figures in the more elaborate method.)

As another example of the use of chi-square we may examine the following figures
of the number of those malaria patients who died and those who recovered, after an
attack of the disease, in two different areas, A and B.   Based on 67 and 29 patients,
the observed mortality rates were 34% and 14% respectively, in the two areas.   Our
purpose is to examine whether this difference could have arisen by chance only.

Table 5.   Distribution of malaria patients according to their
recovery or death, in two areas A and B

	Patients died	Patients recovered	Total number of patients
Area A	23	44	67
Area B	4	25	29
Total	27	69	96

$$\chi^2 = \frac{(23 \times 25 - 44 \times 4)^2 \times 96}{67 \times 29 \times 69 \times 27} = 4.222$$

The value of chi-square is found to be 4.222, which appears significant at the 5 per cent. probability level. Therefore we would conclude, on the basis of 5 per cent. probability level, that our null hypothesis is contradicted and that the mortality rate was different between the regions. There is, however, one important caution to be observed when calculating chi-square based on only small numbers. The test described above has its limitations in that it yields a reliable measure of the probability level of significance only when the expected values in each of the four cells are sufficiently large. Fortunately, however, by means of a simple correction called after the name of F. Yates and termed "correction for continuity", the value is satisfactorily adjusted to take care of small cell values. As a general rule, if the expected number of values in any cell is found to be less than 500, Yates' correction for continuity should be applied. All that is necessary then is to subtract half the total number of observations (e.g. half of 96 in the example given above) from the absolute difference in the two cross-products of cell values as determined in step 1 outlined earlier. The difference of the cross-products is then the corrected difference which is squared and then multiplied by the total number of observations. The product thus obtained is as before divided by the product of the four marginal totals. Thus the corrected chi-square is always smaller than the uncorrected value. The calculation of corrected chi-square for our example is shown below:

$$\chi^2 = \frac{(|23 \times 25 - 44 \times 4| - \frac{96}{2})^2 \times 96}{67 \times 29 \times 69 \times 27}$$

$$= 3.2674$$

The general formula for the corrected χ^2 is:

$$\chi^2 = \frac{(|ad - bc| - \frac{N}{2})^2 N}{(a+b)(c+d)(a+c)(b+d)}$$

As stated earlier only a value of chi-square exceeding 3.841 is to be regarded as statistically significant at the 5 per cent. significance level. Our corrected value of chi-square is now lower than this critical value and hence is not to be considered significant. By the application of an appropriate corrected chi-square test we are led to argue therefore that the difference between the two population groups is not statistically established.

Thus even when the number of observations in individual cells is small the value of corrected chi-square indicates with a fairly reasonable accuracy the probability of the observed results occurring from chance alone. The test is especially useful when the value of chi-square does not fall near critical points such as 3.841 or 6.635. However, in actual practice, especially when dealing with very small numbers, even the corrected chi-square fails to indicate the value of this probability with exactness. In doubtful cases such as for instance when the value of chi-square is found to be near the conventional significance level and the frequencies are very small, it is of interest to know the exact value of the probability that the differences in the two responses could be considered significant from the statistical point of view. A formula for the calculation of exact value of probability is available, but it is beyond the scope of this discussion. (See Fisher, 1950, section 21.02.)

As a caution in the use of X^2 an example may be given where it is sometimes tempting to use it even though it does not provide a valid test.

Suppose 200 children are randomly selected from a large population and examined for spleen enlargement before starting an antimalaria campaign. The spleen rate is found to be 60 per cent. The same children are re-examined some time later after the campaign, and the spleen rate is then found to be 45 per cent. We now want to test whether the decrease in the spleen rate is statistically significant and to judge whether it is attributable to the campaign. The data may be set out in the form of a 2 x 2 table below.

Table 6. Children showing enlargement of spleen before and after an antimalaria campaign

	With enlargement of spleen	With no enlargement of spleen	Total	Percentage
Before the campaign	120	80	200	60%
After the campaign	90	110	200	45%
Total	210	190	400	

The value of X^2 with Yates' correction is:

$$X^2 = \frac{(120 \times 110 - 80 \times 90 - 400/2)^2 \times 400}{210 \times 190 \times 200 \times 200} = 8.43$$

This value is of course highly significant and therefore one may be led to argue on the basis of this test that the effect was significant, and that the campaign had contributed to reduction in the spleen rate.

According to statistical theory, however, the X^2 test for a 2 x 2 table is valid only when the two groups of 200 children are independently selected. In our case the two groups are identical and this method is therefore not valid. The correct method will be to compare the differences observed in the spleen rate between two periods, 60 per cent. and 45 per cent., with some appropriate measure of the degree of fluctuation normally expected in the rate. In other words, we have to know what would have happened if the campaign had not been carried out: would the rate have remained at the same level or increased or decreased? If on the assumption that no antimalaria campaign was carried out we could calculate the probability of the spleen rate of 60 per cent. decreasing by more than 15 per cent. during the period, a statistical test could possibly be made.

Thus the problem is, how the natural fluctuation from one period to another can be evaluated. Of course, the degree of fluctuation would vary from season to season, from year to year, and from village to village. If the pattern of fluctuation is previously known, the observed change in spleen rate could be compared with that figure. However, it will be apparent that we cannot be sure from the above data whether the observed change was caused by sampling variation or by the campaign or was due to seasonal variation peculiar to the village or to a combination of these and possibly other factors.

A method frequently used in such cases is to provide for a control area (see section 4.1). Thus two villages presumably similar may be selected, in one of which an antimalaria campaign is carried out and the other is kept as control.

Measurements on malariometric indices are made before and after the campaign.
Attempts are then made to draw conclusions from these comparisons as to whether the
campaign contributed to the reduction of these rates. However, this procedure again
is not satisfactory because here also we possess no objective evidence that two
villages were really similar and remained so except that one was treated. In this
connexion it is emphasized that an empirical judgement on similarity of conditions
among villages does not always ensure that these villages would remain under
practically similar environmental conditions, before, during, and after the insecticidal operation. Thus it sometimes happens that the spraying of larger doses of
DDT in one village gives significantly inferior results to the spraying of a weaker
solution in another village. Also, even in the same locality, it is not rare that
a mosquito catch in a treated house yields more mosquitos than in an untreated house.

In such observations, the environmental differences among the places under study
are confounded with the possible differences in the efficacy of insecticides.
Differences in anopheline catches or in other malariometric indices should not therefore be taken as the direct indication of differences in toxicity in the insecticides
examined. Due allowance should be made for the possible differences in environmental
conditions among villages or among catching stations.

Granting that such diversity of conditions exist, how can we judge the real
effect of the insecticide? One simple method is to replicate the trial. We first
make a list of all the villages where campaigns are to be carried out and then select
randomly from the list two groups of several villages, one for treatment and the
other for control. Measurements are then compared between two periods and between
two groups. By this means we can be sure, to some extent, that the difference
between groups provides us with a measure of effectiveness of the treatment capable
of being compared with the natural fluctuation. The testing procedure would be as
follows: suppose each of the treated and control areas contains four villages, each
selected at random from a group of 8 villages, the spleen rate is computed from
100 children for each village. Then the difference (spleen rate after campaign) -
(spleen rate before campaign), can be tabulated as follows:

Table 7.   **Difference in spleen rate between two averages**
and two periods

	Treated area	Control area
	-13.2%	+6.3%
	-18.6	-1.8
	-25.1	+0.5
	-15.3	-3.0
Average	-18.05%	+0.50%

We can now test whether the campaign has had any effect in the treated area.   We proceed to test the null hypothesis that the average difference for the treated area is essentially the same as that for the untreated area.   In other words, we are to test whether -18.05% for the treated area is significantly different from +0.50% for the control area.   For this purpose the "t" test explained in section 2.16 can be adopted.

The practical problems involved in planning a suitable field trial are discussed in section 4.3

Contingency tables

The 2 x 2 tabular arrangement discussed earlier is a simple form in which information in respect of two groups can be classified.   Frequently it may be desirable to study the data for each of the two groups in a larger number of categories than two.

For instance, Table 8 below is intended to compare the distribution of spleen sizes in two independent samples of children in the age-group 2-5 years in a WHO Malaria Control Demonstration area in India, before and after DDT spraying operations. The sizes are expressed in class code numbers recommended by Covell et al., 1953.

A tabular presentation such as the following is an example of a "contingency table". Of course, we could have more than two columns as would happen for instance if we were comparing the distribution of spleen sizes at three or more periods, or for three or more places or population groups. The method of analysis described below is of general applicability, i.e. it will apply to tables of any number of columns and rows provided:

(1) the figures in each cell are actual counts (called frequencies) and are not rates or ratios;

(2) no cell contains very small expected frequency, i.e. no cell value for expected frequency is less than about 1;

(3) an independent sample is taken at each time.

In the example given below spleen size 5 contains small numbers, 1 and 0. In such cases we combine the figures with those of the adjacent groups in order to make a group in which the expected frequency is over 1. In this example we consider classes 4 and 5 as one group in the analysis that follows.

Table 8.   Distribution of spleen size before and
after DDT spraying

Class of spleen size	Before spraying	After spraying	Total
0	70	156	226
1	40	89	129
2	150	165	315
3	111	63	174
4	10)11	5)5	15)16
5	1)	0)	1)
Total	382	478	860

There is some indication that after spraying DDT there was a relatively larger number of children with smaller spleen enlargements. Is this difference statistically significant, i.e. are we justified in concluding that this difference is not a mere chance occurrence?

Once again the statistician would begin by postulating the null hypothesis that there is no real difference in the two distributions of children by spleen size, and proceed to test whether the recorded data do or do not contradict his hypothesis. In other words, he will estimate the probability of differences as large as those observed or even larger differences arising from mere chance.

If no real difference existed in the two series, the figures in each row or spleen class should have occurred in the same proportion in all spleen class groups. For instance, out of a total of 860 there were 226 children falling in spleen class zero. Following the simple "rule of three", therefore, we expect $\frac{226}{860}$ x 382 or 100.4 children to fall in the "before spraying" group and $\frac{226}{860}$ x 478 or 125.6 in the "after spraying" category. These then are the expected numbers according to the null hypothesis. The expected numbers "E" falling in each cell, computed as above, are shown below:

Expected cell frequencies

Class of spleen size	Before spraying	After spraying	Total
0	100.4	125.6	226
1	57.3	71.7	129
2	139.9	175.1	315
3	77.3	96.7	174
4 and 5	7.1	8.9	16
Total	382	478	860

As in the case of the calculation of X^2 for a 2 x 2 table, we calculate separately for each cell the quantity $(O - E)^2 \div E$. The quantities thus obtained separately for each cell are then added to give the value of X^2.

$$X^2 = \frac{(70 - 100.4)^2}{100.4} + \frac{(156 - 125.6)^2}{125.6} + \frac{(40 - 57.3)^2}{57.3} + \ldots + \frac{(5 - 8.9)^2}{8.9}$$

$$= 57.54$$

This value of X^2 helps us in judging the validity of the null hypothesis on a probability scale. We cannot judge this X^2 value against the critical level values (3.841 at 5% significance level or 6.635 at 1% significance level) stated earlier which apply only to X^2 calculated from a 2 x 2 table. The reason is that the larger the number of cells the larger will be the expected value of X^2, i.e. the critical level value of X^2 should be related in some way also to the size of the contingency tables (columns and rows). This is done by calculating for each table the "degrees of freedom" which are obtained as the product of one less than the number of columns and one less than the number of rows. A 2 x 2 table, for example, has (2-1)(2-1) or 1 degree of freedom. The above table has (2-1)(5-1) or 4 degrees of freedom. For various degrees of freedom the value of X^2 corresponding to 5% and 1% significance levels are given in Appendix D. From this Appendix it is seen that the critical values of X^2 with 4 degrees of freedom are 9.488 for 5% and 13.277 for 1% level of significance. Our observed value of X^2, i.e. 57.54, exceeds these two critical values. Therefore it is judged to be highly significant.

Values of X^2 at other probability levels of significance will be found in Table IV of Fisher & Yates (1953), page 41.

2.12 Quantitative Measurements

We now consider simple methods for analysing numerical measurements. When the number of such measurements is not very large (less than 50 or so for example), the first step usually taken is to calculate an average value from the individual measurements. Such an average value can be calculated by more than one method, of which the one commonly adopted is to add all the observations and divide by the total number of observations. The value thus obtained is termed the "arithmetical mean". For example, the following measurements of "suspensibility"[1] were obtained on the same sample of DDT by 15 separate tests carried out in the same laboratory:

1.80	1.96	2.00
1.74	1.82	1.95
1.85	1.82	1.97
1.53	1.97	1.93
1.89	1.97	2.10

---

[1] The figures represent the amount in percentage found in suspension 30 minutes after agitating a 2.5% (by weight) DDT suspension prepared from the concentrate, when tested by the method set out in section 8.5 Wld Hlth Org. techn. Rep. Ser. 54.

$$\text{Arithmetical mean} = \frac{1.80 + 1.74 + 1.85 + \ldots + 2.10}{15}$$

$$= \frac{28.30}{15} = 1.887$$

In algebraic symbols, if n is the number of measurements (15 in the present example), and if each individual measurement is denoted by x_1, x_2, x_3, ..., x_n, then arithmetical mean $\bar{x}$ (read as "x bar") is given by:

$$\bar{x} = \frac{x_1 + x_2 + x_3 + \ldots + x_n}{n} = \frac{\Sigma x}{n}$$

The symbol Σ is used, as before, to indicate summation of all the individual values.

If instead of adding all the observations as above, we multiplied them all, we could obtain a "geometric mean" by taking the nth root of the product. Thus, if we had only two observations 1.80 and 1.74 the square root of their product being $\sqrt{1.80 \times 1.74}$ or 1.77 will be the geometric mean. For all the 15 observations given above the geometric mean is obtained by taking the fifteenth root of the product of all values.

$$\text{Geometric mean} = \sqrt[15]{(1.80 \times 1.74 \times 1.85 \ldots \times 2.10)}$$

Its calculation is considerably facilitated by taking logarithms (see Appendix A).

$$\text{Log (geometric mean)} = \frac{1}{15} (\log 1.80 + \log 1.74 + \ldots + \log 2.10)$$

$$= \frac{1}{15} (4.12317) = 0.27488$$

The anti-log of 0.27488 is 1.883 which is the geometric mean.

In algebraic symbols the geometric mean of n observations x_1, x_2, ..., x_n is given by:

$$\text{G.M.} = \sqrt[n]{x_1 \times x_2 \times x_3 \times \ldots x_n}$$

For its calculation we use the relationship:

$$\log (\text{G.M.}) = \frac{1}{n} (\log x_1 + \log x_2 + \ldots + \log x_n) = \frac{1}{n} \Sigma \log x$$

In other words we first find the arithmetic mean of the logarithm of individual measurements and obtain the geometric mean by taking the antilogarithm of such an arithmetic mean.

The use of geometric mean is advisable in preference to arithmetic mean if the series of observations contain one or two abnormally large values. This happens, for instance, in recording parasite counts of individual persons where enormous variation in numerical values is usually encountered, and one infection of very great magnitude may grossly swamp the effect of a large majority of smaller counts. The WHO Drafting Committee (Covell et al., 1953) has suggested the use of the geometric mean in such cases.

Another type of average called the "median" is found by arranging the series of observations either in increasing or decreasing order of magnitude and then picking out the middle one from the series. Thus half the observations fall below the median and half lie above it; the median value thus dividing the series of observations into equal halves. For instance, the above observations when arranged for the highest to the lowest value are as follows: 2.10, 2.00, 1.97, 1.97, 1.97, 1.96, 1.95, 1.93, 1.89, 1.85, 1.82, 1.82, 1.80, 1.74, 1.53.

The eighth value from either end which is the middle value of the series is 1.93. This, therefore, is the median. If the number of measurements is even, then there may be no single mid-value to describe the median. In such a case an average of the two values lying in the middle of the series is regarded as the median.

Another form of average is the "mode" which, as the name itself suggests, describes the general "fashion", being the most frequently occurring value observed in the series. In the above series, for example, the value 1.97 occurs three times, the value 1.82 twice, and the remaining values only once each. The value occurring the largest number of times is 1.97 and will be termed the "mode". The usefulness of mode as a form of average for a small series of observations such as in this example, is doubtful. Its importance lies more in cases where a very large series of observations have been obtained and expressed in the form of a frequency curve. The mode or the modal value will then correspond to the peak of the frequency curve.

Relative advantage or disadvantage of the mean, mode and median. For practical purposes, when the series of observations does not include one or two unduly large measurements, the arithmetic mean is a satisfactory measure of average. If, on the other hand, one or two values included in the series are very large as would happen, for instance, if we were interested in the average duration of hospitalization of malaria patients estimated from a group of 20 patients of whom 18 had been discharged from the hospital within 10 days of their admission, but of whom the remaining two continued to stay in the hospital owing to recurrence of the disease extending over one or two months, the average duration of hospitalization would be a highly inflated figure because of the inclusion of two recurrent cases of the disease. Of course, when we are interested in estimating the amount of medical care needed, the arithmetic mean of the duration of hospitalization for a patient may be a suitable measure for the purpose. On the other hand, when we are interested in knowing the usual duration of malaria hospitalization, a measure markedly influenced by one or two observations is not satisfactory. For this purpose, a median value will be a more satisfactory measure of the average duration of hospitalization than the arithmetic mean. If a very large series of observations were being made, the modal value would also provide in this case a satisfactory measure of the average for our purpose. While the arithmetic mean is considerably affected by unusually large values, and the geometric mean relatively very much less so, the median and mode are unaffected. One disadvantage in the use of geometric mean is that if even one value in the series is zero, the whole product is zero and the geometric mean is zero also. Furthermore, it is not computable when negative values are included in the series.

When individual measurements of a series are not available but have been grouped in the form of a frequency distribution, the value of these various averages can still be obtained by following the same principles. The calculations involved are beyond the scope of this brief introduction. (See Hill, 1955, chapter IV.) The method of calculating the arithmetic mean and median from grouped data may in fact involve less labour than if we were to calculate them from the original series.

2.13 Measures of Variation

Apart from an average value, a feature of considerable importance for study is the degree of variability of individual measurements around its own average.   If all the values included in the series were similar, the mean or one of the values alone could describe the whole experience fairly well.   However, in the above case of suspensibility measures of DDT, the individual measurements vary from 1.53 to 2.10 giving a range of variation of 2.10-1.53 = 0.57.   Since these measurements were all made on the same sample of DDT the range determines the variation arising from sampling errors.   It is not unlikely that in another laboratory a similar series of tests on an identical sample of DDT may have recorded values which did not vary so much among themselves, thus indicating a lower range of experimental errors.

As a simple measure of the variation in the series of figures, the range (difference between the highest and the lowest value) is sometimes used.   However, being based on only two extreme observations and hence ignoring the variability among all the remaining values, the range is generally not regarded as a satisfactory measure of variability of observations, especially when the number of observations is large.   Another defect of the range is that its value becomes greater as the size of observations increases, because more extreme values are expected to arise when a greater number of observations are made.   In recent years the use of the range as a short-cut method in estimating the variance (or standard deviation) of a normal population is becoming popular, because of its simplicity of computation. For further discussion readers are referred to sections 2.6 and 5.6 of Snedecor (1956).

We can study individual variability of each observation from the difference of each observation from the arithmetic mean of the series.   Thus, the first value, namely, 1.80 deviates by (1.80-1.887) or by -0.087, from the arithmetical mean 1.887. The second observation deviates by -0.147 etc.   The 15 deviations of individual measurements from the arithmetical mean are set out below:

-0.087	+0.073	+0.113
-0.147	-0.067	+0.063
-0.037	-0.067	+0.083
-0.357	+0.083	+0.043
+0.003	+0.083	+0.213

If proper regard is paid to the plus and minus signs, the total of all these deviations for the mean value is found to be zero, which should be so since the entire series of observations should balance around the arithmetical mean. A measure of the variability of individual observations around the arithmetical mean cannot therefore be provided by merely taking an algebraic total of these deviations. It can, however, be found by ignoring the minus and plus signs and averaging simply the numerical values. An average of such numerical values of deviations ignoring the signs, gives what is called "mean deviation". In our series of observations

$$\text{Mean deviation} = \frac{.087 + .147 + .037 + \ldots + .213}{15}$$

$$= \frac{1.519}{15} = 0.101$$

In algebraic symbols:

$$\text{Mean deviation} = \frac{\left|x_1 - \bar{x}\right| + \left|x_2 - \bar{x}\right| + \left|x_3 - \bar{x}\right| + \ldots + \left|x_n - \bar{x}\right|}{n}$$

$$= \frac{\sum \left|x - \bar{x}\right|}{n},$$

where n is the number of observations and $\left|x - \bar{x}\right|$ stands for the absolute value of $\left|x - \bar{x}\right|$ without regard to the sign. However, this measure of variability or dispersion is not widely used. More satisfactory measures and the ones most frequently adopted, are what are called the "variance" and the "standard deviation". Their calculation is also based on the deviations of individual values from the arithmetical mean. The deviations are first squared, so that each squared value has the same positive sign. In the example above the following squared deviations are obtained:

.007569	.005329	.012769
.021609	.004489	.003969
.001369	.004489	.006889
.127449	.006889	.001849
.000009	.006889	.045369

The total of these squared deviations when divided by one less than the number of deviations gives a numerical value which is frequently used in statistical analysis and is called the "variance".

Variance = .256933 / 14 = .01835

Algebraically, if V denotes the variance, then

$$V = \frac{(x_1 - \bar{x})^2 + (x_2 - \bar{x})^2 + (x_3 - \bar{x})^2 + \ldots + (x_n - \bar{x})^2}{n - 1}$$

$$= \frac{\Sigma (x - \bar{x})^2}{n - 1}$$

The square root of variance is called "standard deviation". The letter "s" is used to denote standard deviation estimated from a series of observations. It is given by

$$s = \sqrt{\frac{(x_1 - \bar{x})^2 + (x_2 - \bar{x})^2 + \ldots + (x_n - \bar{x})^2}{n - 1}}$$

$$s = \sqrt{\frac{\Sigma (x - \bar{x})^2}{n - 1}}$$

Standard deviation provides us with a measure of the variability on the same scale on which the original observations are given.

Sometimes the symbol σ (sigma) is used in place of the letter s to denote standard deviation. It is customary to designate the value of standard deviation derived from the sample by the letter "s" and to use the symbol σ only for the value theoretically obtained if the entire population was studied. Thus s is a sample estimate of the population value σ, a value that is usually not known.

An easier method of computation which does away with the need of finding the difference of each individual observation from the mean is to use the following relation, which provides the same answer as the formula given above for the standard deviation:

$$s = \sqrt{\frac{\Sigma x^2 - (\Sigma x)^2/n}{n - 1}}$$

The various steps for calculating the standard deviation when this formula is used are:

(i)   square each observation and add, thus obtaining Σx^2;

(ii)   square the total of all measurements and divide by the number of observations. Thus get $(\Sigma x)^2 \div n$. (This quantity is called the "correction term");

(iii)   find the difference between the quantities obtained in steps (i) and (ii) above, i.e. $\Sigma x^2 - \dfrac{(\Sigma x)^2}{n}$

(iv)   divide by n − 1 to obtain the variance;

(v)   take square root and thus obtain the standard deviation.

As an example we may recompute the variance of measurements on the suspensibility data of DDT shown in the last example.

Step   (i) $\Sigma x^2 = 1.80^2 + 1.74^2 + 1.85^2 + \ldots + 2.10^2 = 53.6496$

"   (ii) $(\Sigma x)^2 \div n = (1.80 + 1.74 + 1.85 + \ldots + 2.10)^2 \div 15 = 53.3927$

"   (iii) $\Sigma x^2 - \dfrac{(\Sigma x)^2}{n} = 53.6496 - 53.3927 = 0.2569$

"   (iv) $V = \dfrac{1}{n-1} \left\{ \Sigma x^2 - \dfrac{(\Sigma x)^2}{n} \right\} = \dfrac{0.2569}{14} = 0.01835$

"   (v) $s = \sqrt{V} = \sqrt{0.01835} = 0.135$

The value of the variance is identical to that previously computed.

2.14   Coefficient of Variation

The two statistical measures, namely, arithmetical mean and the standard deviation, are intended to summarize in numerical form two different but important features of a series of measurements. The first provides an estimate of the average value, and the second indicates the extent to which individual observations have a tendency to vary around the average. Both these measures are expressed in the same unit as the original observations.

Generally the variability is expected to be larger in a group with a higher mean than in another group with a lower mean. For instance the variance of height among adults will be greater than the variance among infants, if they are measured on the same scale. A convenient method of comparing variability of these two characteristics is to express each standard deviation as a percentage of the mean. This measure is called the "coefficient of variation".

$$\text{Coefficient of variation} = \frac{\text{Standard deviation}}{\text{Arithmetical mean}} \times 100 = \frac{s}{x} \times 100\%$$

In so far as coefficient of variation is concerned, the original unit of measurement is therefore immaterial.

Sometimes it is of interest to study whether measurements made in terms of one scale are less or more variable than measurements of an altogether different characteristic naturally based on a different scale of units. For instance, let us suppose that measurements of enlarged spleen have been recorded for a group of children. These will show variation in the spleen size. We may also note the ages, heights, body weights, etc. and calculate corresponding arithmetic means and standard deviations. One may well ask whether the variability shown by this group in its spleen size is of the same order of magnitude as the variability in their body weights. The average body weight and the standard deviation of weight measurements will be available in terms of pounds while average spleen size and the variability of individual spleens around the average may be expressed in terms of centimetres. Naturally, pounds and centimetres cannot be compared. In such a case the coefficient of variation could provide a better measure in comparing the variation.

Are children more variable with respect to height or to weight? Coefficients of variation calculated for both height and weight measurements will enable us to make comparisons. Again this coefficient will enable us to study whether a population group is more variable in respect of parasite count or spleen size.

The following data on the length and breadth of wings of Anopheles culicifacies (Rajindar Pal, 1945) illustrate one use of the coefficient of variation:

	Mean (mm)	Standard deviation (mm)
Length of the wing	2.59	0.208
Breadth of the wing	0.622	0.0764

The coefficient of variation of the wing length is computed as

$$\frac{0.208}{2.59} = .0803 \doteq 8\%,$$

while the coefficient of variation of the wing breadth is

$$\frac{0.0764}{0.622} = .1228 \doteq 12\%$$

2.15   Standard Error of the Mean

In the example given earlier of the arithmetical mean, the calculation of the mean was based on 15 measurements.   It is obvious that if we make another series of 15 suspensibility measurements on the same sample of DDT, the values observed may not be identical.   It is also quite likely that the average obtained from the 15 observations of the second series may not be identical with that obtained in the first series.   If the same person were to make a third series of 15 estimations, he may get yet another mean value.   We can theoretically conceive of a very large number of mean values calculated from separate series of individual observations. It would be apparent, of course, that the degree of variability shown by these mean values among themselves would be of a much lower order than the degree of variability shown by individual estimations among themselves provided, of course, the conditions under which estimations were made did not change.

It is known from mathematical theory that if V is the variance of individual observations, and if the mean values are calculated from n observations at a time, then the variance of the series of mean values is given by $\frac{V}{n}$.   Correspondingly, therefore, the standard deviation of the arithmetic means will be $\sqrt{\frac{V}{n}}$, or equal to $\frac{s}{\sqrt{n}}$.

This relationship is helpful because instead of repeating the work of estimating mean values theoretically from an infinitely large number of individual measurements, even a single series of n values can indicate what the range of variation of its mean is likely to be.   In actual cases usually we do not know the exact value of V of the true variance of individual observations and we substitute it with an estimate of V which can be computable from the n observations.   The procedure of computation has already been explained in the previous paragraph.

This quantity $\sqrt{\dfrac{V}{n}}$ is called the "standard error" of the mean.   For instance, this relationship will show that if each mean value is based on four observations, then the variability among the mean values as judged by the standard deviation would be half that shown by individual observations among themselves.   If each mean value is calculated from 100 observations, the arithmetical means will have standard deviation of the order of only one-tenth of the individual observations.

As a numerical example let us compute the standard error of the mean of the measurements of suspensibility given in section 2.11.

$$V = .01835$$

$$\frac{V}{n} = \frac{.01835}{15} = .001223$$

$$\sqrt{\frac{V}{n}} = \sqrt{.001223} = .03497$$

Thus the standard error of the mean in this case is estimated at about .035.

2.16   Comparison of Two Means

Let us suppose that the following 15 measurements were recorded on another sample of DDT in the same laboratory:

2.15	1.98	1.81
2.07	2.04	2.09
2.13	1.99	1.95
2.25	2.17	1.89
2.37	1.98	2.02

T

The arithmetic mean of these observations is 2.059 which is greater than 1.887 found earlier in another series of 15 values. Are these average values significantly different from each other judged from the statistical point of view? Can this difference between 2.059 and 1.887 be attributable to chance variation only? In order to examine this difference, we begin, as before, with the null hypothesis that these two samples have essentially the same suspensibility. A test called the "t" test is available for such a null hypothesis, by which we test the difference between the two means $\bar{x}_1$ and $\bar{x}_2$ against the standard error which a difference is likely to manifest on the basis of our null hypothesis. If the difference $\bar{x}_1 - \bar{x}_2$ actually observed is found to be much greater than its standard error, we judge that our null hypothesis is contradicted by the data, and hence conclude that the difference between the two means is statistically significant.

The variances of the two series are first calculated. Then the standard deviation expected to occur between $\bar{x}_1$ and $\bar{x}_2$ is computed by the formula:

$$\sqrt{\frac{n_1 + n_2}{(n_1 + n_2 - 2)n_1 n_2} \left\{ (n_1 - 1) V_1 + (n_2 - 1) V_2 \right\}},$$

Where n_1 and n_2 are the numbers of observations and V_1 and V_2 the variances of the two series. We then calculate the quantity "t" by dividing the difference between $\bar{x}_1$ and $\bar{x}_2$ by the standard error of the difference.

$$t = \frac{\bar{x}_1 - \bar{x}_2}{\sqrt{\frac{n_1 + n_2}{(n_1 + n_2 - 2)n_1 n_2} \left\{ (n_1 - 1)V_1 + (n_2 - 1)V_2 \right\}}},$$

In the special case where the numbers of observations are equal for the two series $(n_1 = n_2 = n)$, the formula becomes:

$$t = \frac{\bar{x}_1 - \bar{x}_2}{\sqrt{\frac{1}{n}(V_1 + V_2)}}.$$

$$n_1 = n_2 = 15 \text{ and therefore}$$

$$t = \frac{2.059 - 1.887}{\sqrt{\frac{1}{15}(.01835 + .02011)}} = 3.40$$

The larger the absolute value of "t" the weaker is the possibility of the difference arising from chance alone. For assessing the statistical significance, we require to know the value of "t" corresponding to 5% or 1% probability levels of significance. These critical level values of "t" differ according to the number of observations in the two series. The total number of observations in both the series minus two is called the "degree of freedom". In the present case the degrees of freedom are 30-2 or 28. Values of "t" have been published (Fisher & Yates, 1953), for various levels of significance and corresponding to different degrees of freedom. A few values of "t" are given in Appendix E to illustrate the use of this test.

Our value of "t" is -3.40, corresponding to 28 degrees of freedom. It is greater in magnitude than 2.763, the value corresponding to 1% level of significance. It thus indicates that if we assume that our null hypothesis is true there is less than 1% probability of a difference between the two means exceeding the observed value by mere chance. In other words, the difference is to be judged statistically significant.

This test for assessing the difference between the two arithmetic means is of fairly general applicability. The various steps involved in the calculation of the value of "t" are as follows:

1. Find the arithmetic means $\bar{x}_1$ and $\bar{x}_2$ of the two series.

2. Find the variances V_1 and V_2 of the two series.

3. Find the standard error of the difference between the two mean values $\bar{x}_1$ and $\bar{x}_2$ by using the formula:

$$\sqrt{\frac{n_1 + n_2}{(n_1 + n_2 - 2)n_1 n_2} \left\{ (n_1 - 1)V_1 + (n_2 - 1)V_2 \right\}}$$

4.   Divide the difference between the two means by the quantity obtained in step 3, and thus get the value of "t".

5.   Estimate the number of degrees of freedom, which is two less than the total number of observations in the two series, i.e. $n_1 + n_2 - 2$.

The value of "t" is looked up in the "t" table (Fisher & Yates, 1953, see also Appendix E) for the corresponding degrees of freedom, to judge statistical significance of the difference.

2.17   Comparison of Two Variances

Just as the "t" test discussed in the previous section enables us to examine whether two arithmetic means obtained from two different series are statistically different or not, a test called the "F" is available by which the significance of the difference between the two variances V_1 and V_2 can be assessed.   If the two variances are based on n_1 and n_2 observations, the corresponding degrees of freedom are stated to be $n_1 - 1$ and $n_2 - 1$ respectively.   To test whether the two variances are different, we divide the larger variance, say V_1 by the smaller variance V_2 and thus obtain what is called the quantity "F".   The significance of this value is looked up in the tables of "F" values which give for various combinations of $n_1 - 1$ and $n_2 - 1$ the corresponding values of "F" at 5% and 1% levels of significance (Fisher & Yates, 1953, see also Appendix F giving a few selected values of F).

As an example, consider the variances of two series of suspensibility values of DDT given in previous paragraphs, each value being based on 15 observations. In this case:

$$V_1 = .02011$$

$$V_2 = .01835$$

$$n_1 = 15$$

$$n_2 = 15$$

$$F = \frac{V_1}{V_2} = 1.096$$

At the 5% level of significance the value of "F" corresponding to $n_1 - 1 = 14$, $n_2 - 1 = 14$ is 2.84, and at the 1% level of significance the corresponding value of "F" is 3.70 (see Appendix F).   Our value of "F" being lower than even 2.84, shows that the two variances are not to be regarded as different from each other.

2.18   Analysis of Variance

Instead of two series of measurements, we may sometimes have three or more series, and the question may be asked whether the mean values of all the series of observations could be considered to arise from a homogeneous population, or whether among themselves they show statistically significant differences.   The "t" test outlined earlier can enable us to test only two mean values at a time.   Further, this test would not be valid if we were merely to test the difference between the highest and the lowest mean values from among several averages.

A simultaneous comparison of three or more series of observations in respect of their mean values can be made by the technique called "the analysis of variance". Generally speaking, this analysis is based on the idea that if several different series of observations were all to belong to a similar or homogeneous population, then the degrees of variability arising through combining all the observations into a single series would be of about the same order, as shown by any single series of figures separately.   This point will be clear from the following illustration:

Let us suppose that we examine the mean body weight of children at different ages.   If we examined the weights of children belonging only to a single year of age, the individual weights will show a certain degree of variability around the average weight of the series.   If we examine children of the next higher age, their weights separately will also show some variability around the respective average weight. These two variabilities around the respective arithmetic means may be of about the same order, but if we combine the two series into one, the range of variability would naturally be increased for the simple reason that a heterogeneous set of measurements have been put together.   The total variability in the combined series will then be partly due to the natural variation expected among children of the same age, and partly due to the variability attributed to difference in age.   By the technique of analysis of variance the variabilities from these two factors are separately assessed and compared.   If the variability due to age is found to be statistically significantly greater than that around each age, then it is argued that the average weights at the two ages were different.   We can, of course, combine figures at three or more ages and examine whether the variability attributable to age was of a significantly higher order than that found among children considered in separate age-groups.

As an example only of the form in which the results of the analysis of variance are expressed - a form with which malaria workers may get acquainted - we may consider the following illustration:

The same sample of DDT was examined for suspensibility in three different laboratories, two of which made four estimations each, while the third made 12 estimations.   The 20 individual estimations are shown below:

Suspensibility values of DDT from:		
Laboratory A	Laboratory B	Laboratory C
1.36	1.45	1.80
1.35	1.30	1.75
1.47	1.36	1.85
1.49	1.39	1.53
		1.89
		1.96
		1.82
		1.82
		1.97
		1.97
		2.00
		1.95

The three mean values are:

From Laboratory A 1418
From Laboratory B 1375
From Laboratory C 1859

Do the average values of suspensibility found in the three laboratories differ significantly from each other?   The application of the techniques of analysis of variance usually provides an answer in the following tabular form:

Table 9.   Analysis of variance on suspensibility data relating
to tests performed on the same sample of DDT
in three laboratories

	Degrees of freedom	Sum of squares	Mean square	F ratio
Mean Within	2 17	1.02999 0.21859	0.5150 0.0129	F = 39.9
Total	19	1.24858		

There are altogether 20 observations.   The variation around the mean of all the 20 observations (called the "grand mean") is therefore based on 19 degrees of freedom.   The sum of squares of 20 individual deviations around the grand mean is given in the last row of this table as 1.24858.   If, however, we calculate separately the sum of squared deviations of each measurement from the corresponding mean calculated from the measurements made in each laboratory, we would get a total of 0.21859 as the sum of squares, as shown in the third row of this table.   The degrees of freedom contributed by each series will be one less the number of observations in the series, and would therefore be 3, 3, and 11, giving a total of 17.   This provides us with an estimate of what is called the "within variance", or "within mean square", i.e. the variability of individual observations around their own mean values. In the present case it is obtained by dividing 0.21859 by 17.   The value of mean square thus obtained is 0.0129, and is shown in the second row under the heading "mean square".   The variability attributed to the three means is obtained by subtracting the "within sum of squares" from the total sum of the squares.   Thus in our example the sum of squares due to means is: 1.24858 - 0.21859.   This quantity is based on two degrees of freedom, because it relates to three observations.

When this sum of squares is divided by the degrees of freedom, i.e. 2, the mean square due to means is obtained. If the three arithmetic means do not differ significantly from each other, their mean square should be of about the same order of magnitude as the "within variance". In the present example, it is almost 40 times as large as the "within mean square", which according to the F test explained in paragraph 2.18 is judged statistically different. Hence we conclude that three laboratories making suspensibility tests on the same sample of DDT obtained significantly different average values.

An interesting illustration of the technique of analysis of variance is provided by Archibald & Bruce-Chwatt (1956) who compare the average gain in weight in two years among Nigerian schoolchildren, about half of whom were given pyrimethane to suppress malaria, and the others were kept as control. The weight gains in the treated and untreated groups at each year of age were as follows:

Table 10. Weight gains in pounds in treated and untreated groups of Nigerian schoolchildren, January 1953 to December 1954 (Archibald & Bruce-Chwatt's data, 1956)

Age in years	Drug group		Control group	
	Number of children	Mean gain in weight	Number of children	Mean gain in weight
5	51	7.1	33	5.9
6	23	7.7	24	6.7
7	15	9.0	10	7.9
8	18	9.9	21	8.9
9	12	12.0	12	11.1
	119	8.4	100	7.6

The numbers of children on whom each mean gain in weight figure is calculated for individual ages are also shown. For any single age the mean weights could have been compared by the "t" test. But the analysis of variance technique enabled the authors to summarize the results at all ages in the following tabular form of analysis of variance:

Table 11. Analysis of variance of gain in weight

Source of variation	Degrees of freedom	Sum of squares	Mean square	F
Ages ignoring treatment	4	566.34	141.59	
Treatment eliminating ages	1	61.70	61.70	9.81
Error	213	1339.96	6.29	
Total	218	1968.00		

The authors state that: "The value of the F ratio is 9.81 with 1 and 213 degrees of freedom. It exceeds the corresponding critical value at the 1% level of significance, so that the gain in weight is significantly greater for the children in the drug group than for those in the control group."

Another illustration of the use of the analysis of variance technique in malaria work is provided by Viswanathan et al. (1952). They were interested in determining the validity of hand collection of mosquitos on a timed basis for estimating mosquito densities. Six villages in Bombay State were selected, in each of which 12 typical dwellings were chosen as routine collecting stations. These stations were visited by four mosquito collectors at 10 fortnightly intervals. Inasmuch as the variability of the catch could arise because of differences in villages, due to personal efficiency of the investigators, or with the progress of time, it was possible to analyse the variability from each of these factors separately by means of analysis of variance.

The technique of analysis of variance can enable us further not only to study the significance of the difference among means relating to one attribute or factor only, but to several of them at the same time. For instance, we can record measurements of spleen enlargement for children at different ages and by sex. By a single analysis of variance we could then study two separate questions at the same time: (i) whether the mean spleen size differs by sex, and (ii) whether it differs by age.

We could also further test whether there is any differential shift in the spleen size
by age, i.e. if the spleen size varies with age, does it vary in a similar manner for
the two sexes or not?   This is called the "interaction" between two factors, the
existence of which can also be detected at the same time by analysis of variance.
In the same manner, we can examine the variability in a series of measurements arising
from three or more factors.   Such interplay of various factors is frequently noted in
entomological studies as for instance on the species of female anophelines present,
and the temperature and humidity which are known to affect the activity and survival
rates of mosquitos and accordingly also the degree of transmission of malaria in a
locality.   As these vary considerably from season to season and from place to place,
we may have to consider the effect of at least three factors, viz. anopheline species,
temperature and humidity and their interaction on malaria by this technique.   An
interesting application of analysis of variance technique to a study of such inter-
actions is provided by Dakshinamurty (1948).   It is, however, not possible in this
brief discussion to explain the various computational steps necessary for carrying
out analysis of variance.   For further details reference may be made to Snedecor
(1956, Chapters 10 and 11).

2.19   Correlation

It is well known that in many areas malaria epidemics tend to occur after heavy
rainfall.   It is also well known that during and after an epidemic the spleen rate
in the community increases.   In statistical language we then say that a certain
degree of "correlation" exists between malaria and rainfall, or between spleen rate
and malaria.   Between some factors such correlation may be very close, between others
negligible.   What is the degree of this association or correlation?   Can it be
numerically measured?

Correlation theory helps us in estimating the degree to which two or more
variables are associated with each other.   If there is a "high degree of correlation"
i.e. if an increase (or decrease) in one variable is associated with a definite
measurable increase (or decrease) in the other, the existence of correlation may be
obvious.   For instance, if two thermometers calibrated on two different scales of
measurement, e.g. Fahrenheit and Centigrade are both dipped in a fluid and the
temperature varied, the increase or decrease in the temperature of one thermometer

would correspond in almost exact proportion with an increase or decrease in the other, so much so that knowing the reading of one thermometer at any instant, we could state almost with certainty what the reading was in the other.   This, of course, is an ideal case or a case of "perfect correlation", but such cases in malaria studies are rare.   We can think of different areas in some of which malaria incidence and rainfall may be highly correlated, and others in which a high rainfall may be followed by a decrease in the incidence of malaria.   Such an association is termed "negative correlation", which implies that an increase in one variable is associated with a corresponding decrease in the other.   The term "positive correlation" is used to denote association when an increase in one variable corresponds to an increase in the other, and decrease is associated with decrease.   We can also conceive of areas in which no association may exist between rainfall and malaria.

For the purpose of measuring the degree of association, it is customary to calculate what is called the "coefficient of correlation".   The value of the correlation coefficient is 1.0 in the case of a perfect positive correlation.   If no association whatsoever exists between two values, the coefficient of correlation is zero.   The range of the coefficient is thus from +1 to -1, but as a measure of the absolute intensity of association the nearer the value is to ± 1 the higher is the degree of association.   If, for instance, in one area the coefficient of correlation between rainfall and malaria is of the order of 0.8 and in another only 0.2, we say that rainfall is more highly associated with malaria in the former area than in the latter.   Furthermore, if in one area the coefficient of correlation between these two variables is +0.8 and in another -0.8, we say that the degree to which the variables are correlated with each other is the same in both areas, but that in one area the association is of positive and in another of a negative kind.   The coefficient of correlation thus enables us to express by means of a single numerical figure the degree of association existing between two factors as well as to understand whether that association is of a positive or a negative kind.   This coefficient thus provides a measure not only for studying the existence of association but also for comparing the degree of correlation between different sets of factors.

It must be noted, however, that the existence of correlation between any two factors does not necessarily imply a cause-and-effect relationship. The numerical value of the coefficient of correlation merely indicates that any change in one factor corresponds with a change in the other. Of course, some factors may be related in such manner that one is the cause of the other, as for instance, we have reason to believe that an increase in malaria incidence is the cause of a rise in the spleen rate. But sometimes two factors may show similar variation without one being directly dependent on the other: the correlation occurring perhaps because yet another factor was responsible for variation in both of them. As an example, it may be found that in a certain country malaria incidence is highly correlated with the density of population, i.e. the incidence rate of the disease is generally high in densely-populated regions and low in sparsely-populated regions. By establishing a numerically high degree of correlation we cannot, of course, argue in this case that high density of population is the result of high malaria incidence rate or vice versa. Quite likely the population may be dense because of proximity to water, so that it is the presence of large numbers of breeding places in or around densely-populated areas that may in reality be responsible for high malaria incidence. Again, it may be found that the density of population is highly negatively correlated with the case fatality rate of malaria, i.e. per 100 malaria cases more may be dying in less-densely-populated regions than in more-densely-populated places. The real explanation of this may be the availability of better facilities for the treatment of malaria cases in large heavily-populated areas. It is not uncommon in statistical studies on correlation to come across instances when an unwary investigator is tempted to interpret the existence of high correlation between two factors as proof of cause-and-effect relationship. Such misinterpretations generally occur when studying time series, i.e. figures recorded over a long period of time. As a concrete example, if we study annual figures of the number of radio sets in use by a population, we may find a gradual increase with the progress of time. For the same population we may find a steady decrease from year to year in the incidence of malaria deaths. The two series of figures would then show a high degree of negative correlation which of course may indicate or establish nothing. Existence of correlation, therefore, should not be confused with causation. The task of the investigator is not to accept the value of the coefficient of correlation on its face value, but to try and secure satisfactory proof or disproof of cause-and-effect relationship if a significant degree of positive or negative correlation is found to exist.

The first step in the study of this degree of association between two variables is to prepare what is called a "dot" or "scatter" diagram. Figure 19 gives examples of such a diagram, which are based on observations shown in Table 12. The data relate to annual malaria incidence in the Punjab, India, measured by means of epidemic figure[1] (x) and spleen rates measured in the month of November, i.e. following the seasonal rise of malaria (y), and in the month of June, i.e. prior to the onset of the malaria season (z), for a series of years (Yacob & Swaroop, 1947).

It might be noted here that in general the correlation coefficient measures the degree to which the dots assemble around a line that is straight and not curved. When the dots assemble along a curved course the correlation coefficient will not be close to 1.0 or -1.0. In other words this coefficient is not a suitable measure of a curvilinear relationship between two variables. It is therefore necessary first to ascertain whether the spot diagram in question shows more or less a straight line relationship so that the computation of the correlation coefficient is justifiable.

In algebraic symbols the coefficient of correlation is defined by the following formula for a series of pairs of observations (x_1, y_1), (x_2, y_2), (x_n, y_n):

$$r = \frac{\Sigma\ (x_i - \bar{x})(y_i - \bar{y})}{\sqrt{\Sigma\ (x_i - \bar{x})^2\ \Sigma\ (y_i - \bar{y})^2}},$$

where $\bar{x}$ and $\bar{y}$ are arithmetic means of x and y, respectively:

$$\bar{x} = \frac{1}{n}\ (x_1 + x_2 + \ldots + x_n)\ = \frac{1}{n}\ \Sigma\ x_i$$

$$\bar{y} = \frac{1}{n}\ (y_1 + y_2 + \ldots + y_n)\ = \frac{1}{n}\ \Sigma\ y_i.$$

The computation is easier if the following formula is used:

$$r = \frac{\Sigma\ x_i y_i - \frac{1}{n}(\Sigma x_i)(\Sigma y_i)}{\sqrt{\left\{\Sigma\ x_i^2 - \frac{(\Sigma\ x_i)^2}{n}\right\}\left\{\Sigma\ y_i^2 - \frac{(\Sigma y_i)^2}{n}\right\}}},$$

which can be shown to be equivalent to the formula given above.

---

[1] The "epidemic figure" in this example was computed by dividing the average monthly fever mortality from October to December by the corresponding average of the previous four months of April to July of each year (see paragraph 4.4.3)

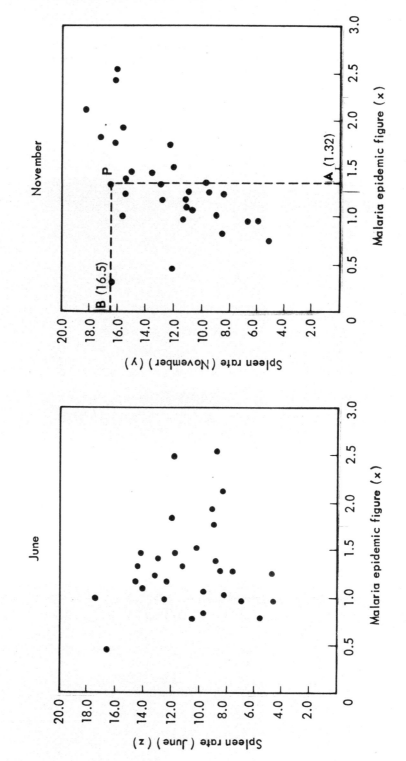

Fig. 19 Punjab, India. «Scatter» or «dot» diagram showing the relationship between rainfall and spleen rate in the months of June and November, 1914-1943

WHO 7323

Table 12.   Punjab, India.   Epidemic figure and spleen rate estimated in the months of June and November 1914-1943

Year	Malaria epidemic figure	Spleen rate (%)	
		Month of November i.e. after the malaria season	Month of June i.e. prior to the malaria season
	(x)	(y)	(z)
1914	1.32	16.5	14.5
1915	1.10	11.1	14.2
1916	1.76	12.4	9.1
1917	2.46	16.2	11.9
1918	0.47	12.3	16.7
1919	1.51	12.1	10.2
1920	0.83	8.7	9.8
1921	1.28	11.1	8.4
1922	1.38	9.8	8.7
1923	1.93	15.7	9.0
1924	1.49	15.1	11.8
1925	1.40	15.5	13.0
1926	1.83	17.3	12.0
1927	1.00	15.8	17.4
1928	0.99	11.4	12.6
1929	1.79	16.3	10.6
1930	1.23	15.6	13.2
1931	1.33	13.0	11.3
1932	1.16	11.1	12.3
1933	2.11	18.5	8.3
1934	1.17	12.8	14.4
1935	1.07	10.8	9.8
1936	1.01	9.2	8.2
1937	0.97	6.7	7.0
1938	0.79	5.3	5.4
1939	0.98	6.0	4.6
1940	1.25	8.5	4.7
1941	1.28	9.5	7.5
1942	2.54	16.2	8.7
1943	1.48	13.6	14.2

As a numerical example let us compute the coefficient of correlation, according to the latter formula, between epidemic figures (series marked x) and November spleen rate (series marked y) in the foregoing Table 12.

Step I: $\Sigma\, x_i y_i$

Find the product of each pair of observations and add the products.

Thus find: $(1.32 \times 16.5)+(1.10 \times 11.1)+\ldots+(1.48 \times 13.6)$

$= 21.780 + 12.210 +\ldots+ 20.128 = 541.933$

Step II: $\frac{1}{n}\,(\Sigma\, x_i)(\Sigma\, y_i)$

Multiply the two totals of the series x and y, and then divide this product by the number of observations.

$\Sigma\, x_i = 40.91, \quad \Sigma y_i = 374.1, \quad n = 30$

Therefore $\frac{1}{30} \times 40.91 \times 374.1 = 510.148$

Step III: Find $\Sigma\, x_i y_i - \frac{1}{n}\,(\Sigma\, x_i)(\Sigma\, y_i) = $ Numerator

Subtract the quantity obtained in Step II from that found in Step I.

$541.933 - 510.148 = 31.785$

Step IV: $\Sigma\, x_i^2$

Square individual values of x and add them.

$1.32^2 + 1.10^2 +\ldots+ 1.48^2 = 1.7424 + 1.2100 +\ldots+ 2.1904$

$= 62.2541$

Step V: $\frac{1}{n}\,(\Sigma\, x_i)^2$

The correction term for the sum of squares of x.

$\frac{1}{30} \times 40.91^2 = 55.7876$

Step VI: $\Sigma\, y_i^2$

Same as Step IV but with y.

$16.5^2 + 11.1^2 +\ldots+ 13.6^2 = 272.25 + 123.21 +\ldots+ 184.96$

$= 5025.45$

Step VII: $\qquad \frac{1}{n}\left(\Sigma y_1\right)^2$

Same as Step V but with y.

$$\frac{1}{30} \times 374.1^2 = 4665.03$$

Step VIII: $\qquad \sqrt{\left\{\Sigma x_1^2 - \frac{1}{n}\left(\Sigma x_1\right)^2\right\}\left\{\Sigma y_1^2 - \frac{1}{n}\left(\Sigma y_1\right)^2\right\}} = \text{Denominator}$

Substituting numerical values obtained in Steps IV to VII we get

$$\sqrt{\left\{62.2541 - 55.7876\right\} \times \left\{5025.45 - 4665.03\right\}} = \sqrt{6.4665 \times 360.42}$$

$$= 2330.7 \qquad = 48.277$$

Step IX: $\qquad r = \dfrac{\Sigma x_1 y_1 - \frac{1}{n}\left(\Sigma x_1\right)\left(\Sigma y_1\right)}{\sqrt{\left\{\Sigma x_1^2 - \frac{1}{n}\left(\Sigma x_1\right)^2\right\}\left\{\Sigma y_1^2 - \frac{1}{n}\left(\Sigma y_1\right)^2\right\}}}$

Divide the quantity obtained in Step III by the quantity obtained in Step VIII.

$$r = \frac{31.785}{48.277} = 0.658$$

The coefficient of correlation between malaria epidemic figure and November spleen rate is thus found to be 0.658.

In the same manner the coefficient of correlation between malaria epidemic figure and spleen rate in the month of June will be found to be -0.105.

It is of course to be understood that when dealing with two variable factors, even if in reality there is no association between them, the value of the coefficient of correlation will not necessarily be absolutely zero, i.e. insignificantly small positive or negative values of the coefficient may nevertheless be obtained owing to chance factors. As a rough method of judging whether the observed value of the coefficient of correlation possesses statistical significance, we may use the following simple rule in cases where the number of pairs of values is large, i.e. about 30 or more.

Multiply the coefficient of correlation by the square root of the number of pairs. If this multiplication reaches a figure exceeding 2, the value of the coefficient of correlation is most probably significant.

For instance, in the above example, the coefficient of correlation between the malaria epidemic figure and spleen rate in the month of November is found to be 0.658.   The number of pairs of observations is 30.   Therefore we calculate 0.658 x$\sqrt{30}$ = 3.56, a figure exceeding 2 and hence regarded as statistically indicating the existence of association.   While this simple method will provide an indication of whether the value emerges into statistical significance, more rigorous methods are available to establish it (Fisher, 1950).

The following values of the coefficient of correlation (or the values exceeding them) are to be considered statistically significant at the 5% or the 1% level of significance (Fisher & Yates, 1953).

Table 13.   Values of the coefficient of correlation significant at 5% and 1% probability level of significance

Number of pairs of values	Value of the coefficient of correlation significant at probability level of:	
	5%	1%
4	0.95	0.99
5	0.88	0.96
10	0.63	0.76
20	0.44	0.56
30	0.36	0.46
50	0.28	0.36
100	0.20	0.26
500	0.09	0.12
1000	0.06	0.08

By way of illustrating the uses to which the correlation technique can be put in malaria work we may quote the following interesting examples:

Even though it is known that in some localities epidemics of malaria follow heavy rainfall, can this information be made the basis of predicting the magnitude of malaria outbreaks from a foreknowledge of rainfall in the locality?   If so, how early can such a prediction be made?   In this connexion the data in respect of one district in North India, viz. Hissar, may be quoted.   It was known from past

experience that epidemics of malaria broke out during the months of August and
September in that district. The magnitude of malaria mortality was first calculated
for each year by means of an annual epidemic figure. The rainfall figure for each
individual month prior to this period was then correlated with the annual epidemic
figures during the period 1914-1943. The following coefficients of correlation
were obtained:

Table 14. Coefficient of correlation between monthly rainfall and
epidemic figure, Hissar District, 1914-1943

Rainfall in the month of:	Coefficient of correlation between monthly rainfall and epidemic figure
January	-0.06
February	0.01
March	-0.15
April	0.46
May	0.10
June	0.11
July	0.17
August	0.53
September	0.39
October	0.14

The high value of the coefficient of correlation for the months of August and
September merely indicates that increased rainfall in malaria season aggravates the
disease. But what is of greater value is the fact that the coefficient of
correlation between malaria and the rainfall about five months earlier (April) is
also high. A study like this reveals the possibility of using the April rainfall
as a basis for predicting the occurrence of malaria epidemics in Hissar District
some four or five months in advance.

Could the spleen data collected routinely for the district also be made on the
basis of such a prediction? Spleen censuses were carried out each year in Hissar
District during the months of June and November. The coefficient of correlation
between pairs of values of spleen rate in June and November and epidemic figure
during the period 1914-1943 were found to be -0.19 and +0.47 respectively.

The latter figure, indicating positive correlation, is understandable because a rise in spleen rate is expected to occur subsequent to a malaria outbreak. The coefficient of correlation between spleen rate in June, i.e. before the malaria season, and the epidemic figure is statistically very low, thus providing no basis for prediction.

Viswanathan et al. (1952) provide another illustration of the use of the coefficient of correlation. They were interested in determining whether mosquito catches made on the basis of "per man-hour" were an adequate indication of the total mosquito population resting in the place at the time of collection. For this purpose, the resting mosquitos were collected first by hand with a collection tube and flash-light for exactly 30 minutes in each station, and subsequently the rooms were sprayed with pyrethrum extract, and the knocked down mosquitos were collected from specially placed white ground-sheets. Altogether 620 separate observations were made, providing 620 pairs of values of hand catches and pyrethrum-killed mosquitos. The coefficient of correlation between these two series of values was found to be 0.36. The coefficient of correlation between the hand catch and the total catch is positive and even though statistically significant is not high in value. While therefore it can be concluded that if the hand catch is high, the population of mosquitos is also high, it is doubtful whether a sufficiently reliable estimate of the latter population can be made on the basis of hand captures. This is because the statistical error of this estimate will still be high.

2.20 Sampling

Surveys of human population may be carried out either by examining every individual in the population or only a sample of it. For populations of large size, the former method is generally not expedient because of the prohibitive cost involved, the unavailability of adequate numbers of trained staff and the long waiting period before the entire mass of statistics can be analysed. On the other hand, when the need exists for quick but elaborate information on various items at frequent intervals, the use of sampling technique is to be preferred. It has been found in practice that whenever information is not needed on all the individual sections or communities into which the population can be divided, we can obtain more accurate information for the entire population with a few reliable trained investigators working on a properly selected sample of the population than would be possible by a large team of untrained investigators employed on a full-scale survey.   There are of course certain items of information which cannot be obtained from an examination of a sample, but then we must balance the probable inaccuracy of the sample against the economies effected. The error associated with an estimate obtained from a sample can be calculated by means of formulae and we can then decide whether we are prepared to accept such an error or not.   For this reason, in almost all branches of statistical studies on human populations, sampling procedures are gradually replacing complete surveys. In the recent past, considerations of accuracy and of keeping down the cost, have led to rapid advances in the technique of sampling and in the standardization of methods and terminology.   Considerable interest in this matter has been shown at the international level by the United Nations through its Sub-Commission on Statistical Sampling.

Briefly stated, the object of modern sampling techniques is to obtain the maximum accuracy or precision of information for the labour and money expended. In other words, it aims at a desirable precision of the results with the minimum labour and money.   Modern sampling techniques provide usable information about the characteristics of a large group of people quickly and moderately cheaply. It is true that any estimate made from a sample is subject to error;   what is equally true is that any estimate made from a survey of the entire population is also subject to error.   There are many other sources from which errors may arise such as, for instance, errors from non-response, errors in measurement, errors in the preparation of estimates, and errors due to the fact that the population characteristics change with time, etc.

The sort of problems in which the application of sampling is justified in malaria work or health work in general, include: the obtaining of information about the prevalence of malaria (morbidity rate, parasite rate, spleen rate, etc.) or of the level of health of persons living in an area, evaluating periodically the results of malaria control or other health procedures; the obtaining and extraction of information from a large mass of data and the evaluation of the reliability or completeness of any recording system.

The manner in which a sample is selected influences only one component of the error and not the whole. A survey may of course be ruined because of poor selection of sample, but it may also be ruined even if the sample has been well selected. The need for constant care at all stages of the survey is therefore emphasized, and it is recommended that the points at which any projected survey will be most vulnerable should be foreseen. Experience has shown that it may pay to take a relatively small sample in order to have the resources concentrated on the reduction of some other sources of error, such as those arising from non-response or errors in measurement.

All the same, the need for a good sample design is imperative. A good sample must satisfy the following criteria:

(a) Following the familiar economic maxim that one should get the most for one's money, we should try to select that sample which will provide the desired degree of precision as cheaply as possible. In other words, if the amount of funds available for the survey is specified, the design should yield the highest degree of accuracy. In this connexion the first question that must be answered is: how small do we want this sampling error to be? This, of course, is related to the question: how precise would we like the estimate to be? This question is usually answered by specifying the standard error (σ sigma) which we wish our estimate to have. (The term "standard error" was explained in section 2.15.) From the theory of probability we expect our estimate not to vary beyond $\pm 2\sigma$ in more than 5% of cases. The specification of the standard error should be made by the person who proposes to use the results of this survey and should depend on the precision needed for such use. While a decision for a large standard error may diminish the utility of results, it is necessary to remember that a demand for unnecessarily high precision may only involve a waste of resources. In deciding the size of sampling error at which we wish to aim, account should also be taken of the magnitude of errors arising from other sources. For instance, if we wish to estimate the spleen rate in a population correctly to within $\pm 10\%$, and therefore choose a sampling standard error of $\pm 5\%$, we should be sure that other errors likely to arise in this estimation, such as the personal error of the investigator, are not likely to exceed 10%. There is no point in having a very small sampling error if other errors still make the estimate imprecise.

(b)   The sample design must itself provide an estimate of the sampling error. This is possible only when a certain degree of random selection is introduced in the sampling procedure.   When the condition of random selection is satisfied the sampling error can be estimated by using a suitable formula deduced by the theory of probability.

(c)   The design should be practicable, i.e. capable of being carried out in practice - sample theory and sample practice must be compatible.

2.20.1   Random samples

An easy, and the most commonly employed, method of drawing a sample is the method of "simple random sampling" in which rules of chance alone decide which of the individual units in the population are to be chosen.   This method satisfies the condition that it gives every unit in the population an equal chance of being included in the sample.   The general procedure is as follows.   Firstly, we need a sub-division of the population into "sampling units".   Thus, for instance, when a spleen survey is to be carried out we would consider each individual person as constituting a separate sampling unit.   In some surveys the sampling unit may be a household or even a village.   For purposes of simple random sampling, these units are first serially numbered and then the desired proportion or probability of inclusion is decided upon.   For instance, we may desire to take a sample of 1 in 10, 1 in 20 or so on.   Then, a simple method which can be adopted for drawing a random sample is that for each sampling unit a separate card is prepared bearing its serial number and the pack of cards is thoroughly shuffled.   As many cards are pulled at random out of this pack as the number of units we require to include in the sample.   The cards, thoroughly mixed, have all equal chances of being included in this sample, and since each card corresponds to a sampling unit in the population, the draw provides a random sample of the entire population under study.

This procedure is cumbersome and work is much facilitated by reference to a table of random numbers (see Appendix B).   In this Appendix the numbers are all arranged in a random manner.   There are eight columns and seven rows of groups of five digits.   The property of this list is that whichever way one reads these digits, horizontally or vertically, the order of the digits will be found to be random. This applies not only to the reading of single digits but to groups of two together or to groups of three together, and so on.   The following example will explain their use.

In the simplest case, let us suppose that we wish to draw a random sample of four children out of nine who, in a serial list, bear numbers 1 to 9. Take any column, say the first, and read 1, so the first child falls in the sample. Reading vertically, the next child included in the sample is the one bearing serial number 6. So, also, we include the one bearing number 5. The next digit in the table is again 6, but since this child has already been included in the sample, we skip this digit and take the next, viz. 3. Thus the four children included in the sample are those bearing serial numbers 1, 6, 5 and 3.

Following the same procedure, if five children were to be included we should also take the child bearing serial number 9.

If we were sampling out of a total of 10 children, the digit 0 in the table of random numbers will refer to the child bearing serial number 10.

If the number of sampling units is greater than 10, then we use two columns together of the table of random numbers.

Let us suppose that out of 80 villages which have been listed in serial order we wish to select 10 villages at random. For the purpose of selecting 10 random serial numbers, none of which should exceed 80 because we have only 80 villages to choose from, we can begin reading groups of two numbers from anywhere in this table, i.e. beginning from any column or row of the table. For instance, let us say that we place our finger at random on the table and let us say that it falls on the third column and fourth row of the group which contains the digits 24705. We could then proceed vertically downwards reading the first two digits which would correspond to the serial number of villages to be selected at random. Thus we will select numbers 24 and 15. Next we come to digit 92 which exceeds the highest serial number of available villages and is therefore ignored. The next serial number of village to be included in the random sample will then be 68, followed by 25 and 1. Since the next number is again 25 which has already been included, this number is ignored and we pass on to numbers 63, 10, 5, 69 and 41. These are therefore the serial numbers of 10 villages selected at random out of the 80 available. Rearranged in increasing order they are: 1, 5, 10, 15, 24, 25, 41, 63, 68 and 69. We could just as well have proceeded horizontally, and looking at groups of two digits together could have thus selected instead, beginning from the same point, the serial numbers 24, 70, 53, 47, 12, 70, 18, 30, 31 and 55. Any number which appears twice is written only once and any number exceeding the maximum number to be chosen is ignored.

The digits 00 are identified with serial number 100 in order to make sure that serial number 100 has an equal chance of being included in the sample.

If our complete serial list contained more than 99 but not exceeding 1000 items, then for the purpose of random selection we should consider groups of three digits together.

Suppose 10 families are to be selected out of a total of 650. We may consider the first three columns of the table and read 103, 623 and 576. Then we come to 670, a figure exceeding our total number and therefore to be ignored. The other seven numbers included in the sample are 362, 558, 9, 107, 49, 431 and 522. Rearranged in increasing order our sample will comprise serial numbers 9, 49, 103, 107, 362, 431, 522, 558, 576, 623.

Other ways of using the table are explained below.

To select at random 10 families out of a list of 190. This can be done as before by taking three columns and discarding any number exceeding 190. But this would mean discarding about five numbers out of every six. In order to avoid this unnecessary work, we proceed first as follows:

```
200 is subtracted from numbers between 201 and 400
400  "          "       "       "      401  "  600
600  "          "       "       "      601  "  800
800  "          "       "       "      801  "  999
```

Note: 00 will count as 200

The first three columns will then provide random numbers as follows:

Random number	Converted number
103	103
623 (-600)	23
576 (-400)	176
670 (-600)	70
362 (-200)	162

and so on.

As a convenient and general rule for selecting random numbers from a total figure lying between

(a) 101 and 200 subtract multiples of 200 as shown in the example;

(b) 201 and 300 subtract 300 from random numbers between 301 and 600
      subtract 600 from random numbers between 601 and 900
      discarding all numbers above 900;

(c) 301 and 500 subtract 500 from random numbers in the table which exceed
      500, regarding 000 as 500.

If the number of items to be selected is more than half the total number of items, it would be more convenient to draw a sample first of those which should not be included in the sample.

Even though the table of random numbers used in the manner explained above will greatly facilitate the selection of random samples, it may nevertheless not be easy for unskilled field staff to use the tables. Special tables can easily be prepared in advance which would give the desired sets of random allocation or selection in increasing order and covering the most likely situations. As an illustration, let us suppose that the total number of sampling units is likely to lie between 401 and 500, and that we are always to draw a sample of 100 units. A list of 100 such random numbers is given in Table 15. These numbers are arranged in increasing order. In actual practice, when selecting such numbers it should be borne in mind that some units selected may have to be excluded for reasons beyond control, e.g. willingness to co-operate or absence of the persons. To cover such cases, additional numbers should be selected to make provision for figures between the total number of families in the list and 500. Forty supplementary numbers are also given in the table. Whenever a selected unit refuses to co-operate, is absent, or the number is higher than the total number in the list, we include one of these supplementary numbers, always starting from the top of the first column. Thus, if the list contains 458 units, then the six numbers 461, 468, 477, 492, 494 and 498, should be replaced by 199, 351, 121, 373, 227 and 47.

Table 15.   Selection of 100 random numbers from a population
of about 500 in size

100 random numbers					Additional numbers	
3	112	181	274	382	199	87
23	123	183	276	387	351	211
33	125	185	277	402	121	59
34	128	186	285	409	373	394
38	130	187	294	410	227	200
50	141	193	299	412	47	369
51	146	202	307	413	137	428
52	147	204	311	417	157	65
55	149	210	315	424	365	469
57	159	217	316	430	296	384
66	160	218	319	443	442	495
76	162	225	324	456	165	72
79	163	234	332	457	250	286
80	166	237	342	458	363	441
82	167	288	344	461	414	341
84	169	240	345	468	171	329
86	175	243	352	477	239	9
94	176	245	356	492	206	333
97	178	266	377	494	358	403
102	180	269	378	498	155	2

The drawing of a random sample is thus based on the availability of a list of the sampling units in the population.   But such lists as are often found may be incomplete or involve duplication or contain inaccurate information, despite the most authoritative assurances to the contrary.   A revision of the list and its completion would, therefore, in every case be necessary to ensure that no sampling unit is missed.   In the absence of such a list, one should be compiled, even if it is found to be expensive and time consuming.   This is usually done at the time a census of the population is being carried out in connexion with the preliminary malaria survey.   In connexion with malaria demonstration work, we would require such lists of households and individuals.   These lists could, of course, be prepared simultaneously.

A population can be thought of as constituting various types of sampling units, such as villages or towns, blocks of houses, families or individual persons. Which of these units should be chosen as the basis of sampling? For some studies, of course, the sampling unit will be the individual as, for instance, for determining spleen rate or parasite rate in a village. But for other purposes, such as testing the costs involved in insecticide spraying, a house or a block of houses may form an appropriate unit. The choice of the sampling unit is determined by the consideration of securing the maximum precision in the information for a given cost subject, of course, to the practical convenience of field work.

2.20.2 Random sampling from sprayed surfaces

In connexion with tests on the sorption of DDT by sprayed surfaces, it may be necessary to take samples of, say, 5 cm^2 surface from a larger sprayed surface. These samples should be drawn at random. The procedure of drawing such samples is as follows:

Suppose the sprayed surface is square in shape, each side being 1 m. In order to draw a random sample we first choose pairs of random numbers, each number being less than 100 cm. In such a pair, the first random number will correspond to the abscissa value (x), i.e. the co-ordinate along the horizontal axis is measured from the origin. The origin will be the bottom left-hand corner of the sprayed surface. The second value of the pair will correspond to the ordinate (y). A number of pairs of xy values are shown in Table 16. For the purpose, therefore, of drawing a random sample on a square metre surface all that is necessary is to pick out any pair of xy values from this table. Then, beginning from the bottom left-hand corner of the one square metre surface, we measure horizontally a distance in centimetres equal to the chosen value of x. Starting from that point on the horizontal axis we then move up by y cm. The point thus obtained is the one which localizes at random the middle point of the 5 cm^2 sample. For example, if we chose the first pair of xy values in this table, namely, x = 10 cm, y = 27 cm, we measure along the horizontal axis 10 cm from the bottom left-hand corner. From this point we measure 27 cm vertically, thus obtaining the random point.

This table provides 200 pairs of xy values corresponding to the possibility of selecting 200 points at random on a one square metre surface. In making random selection it is immaterial which pairs of values are chosen, i.e. we may choose the pair of xy values from any column or row. If it is found that any two samples overlap - which is likely to happen if the random points fall very near each other - then only one of the two should be selected. The table has been so constructed that in any block of five points no overlapping should arise.

If it happens that the sprayed surface is not a square in shape but is rectangular, then Table 17 can be used to cover the case where no side of the rectangle exceeds 1.5 m. The method of selecting the random points on the surface is the same as explained above. If any random point chosen from this table happens to fall outside the area of the sprayed surface, then the next pair of values should be taken and so on.

2.20.3   Methods of sampling

The drawing of a simple random sample is the basis of all good sampling techniques. For different frameworks of the survey, however, certain variations or improvements in technique can be introduced particularly when some prior information is available regarding the variability amongst the individual sampling units of the population. The aim of these modifications in sampling procedures is to increase the accuracy for any given cost and such techniques as stratification, sampling by stages (multi-stage sampling), systematic sampling, and what is called the multi-phase sampling, are used. A brief account of these techniques is given below. For more detailed discussion of sampling methods reference may be made to F. Yates (1953).

When we postulate in advance the size of the sampling error which we are willing to accept and then select the sample so that our statistical conclusions about the characteristics of the whole will not have a sampling error greater than the one we have accepted, we are engaged in what is usually called "probability sampling" (USA, 1954). The word "chunk" has been used to denote a sample, the selection of which is dictated primarily by convenience or by administrative considerations and

Table 16.   Random points (x, y) in cm for sampling from square surface
of side 1 metre

x	y	x	y	x	y	x	y	x	y
10,	27	42,	88	25,	62	63,	61	8,	86
28,	41	77,	94	63,	19	68,	96	39,	14
34,	21	78,	83	18,	66	87,	83	30,	49
61,	81	87,	76	63,	48	49,	52	41,	28
61,	15	91,	43	13,	27	80,	62	23,	56
91,	76	84,	97	89,	95	32,	84	55,	7
36,	46	67,	63	96,	82	85,	39	51,	14
4,	37	96,	23	10,	5	97,	5	3,	42
63,	62	61,	88	5,	39	75,	89	44,	22
78,	47	23,	23	76,	16	9,	18	85,	13
87,	68	13,	54	61,	81	84,	8	3,	61
47,	60	86,	57	96,	47	79,	26	48,	38
56,	88	8,	6	72,	73	46,	68	6,	19
31,	54	34,	94	76,	83	28,	10	55,	58
68,	12	60,	50	71,	50	94,	11	86,	30
63,	29	87,	21	76,	51	43,	63	96,	94
45,	65	34,	41	59,	19	55,	78	14,	82
39,	65	53,	90	82,	82	9,	62	60,	59
73,	71	15,	43	16,	86	44,	88	63,	21
72,	20	10,	77	44,	91	36,	23	89,	17
67,	22	59,	41	37,	30	20,	18	7,	41
37,	48	86,	67	75,	20	97,	48	95,	24
68,	8	13,	17	65,	95	54,	8	65,	72
14,	23	43,	36	94,	21	26,	88	7,	80
49,	8	66,	50	34,	41	32,	97	54,	31
78,	37	26,	51	53,	14	59,	85	83,	36
37,	21	63,	70	88,	59	27,	77	80,	30
14,	29	16,	4	65,	28	42,	94	39,	68
58,	43	20,	11	73,	43	24,	17	90,	74
10,	43	82,	29	48,	62	76,	58	75,	31
44,	38	80,	72	28,	97	45,	71	53,	56
90,	69	74,	13	76,	96	59,	25	78,	91
41,	47	21,	44	79,	57	11,	52	93,	62
91,	94	8,	43	29,	18	67,	53	47,	97
80,	6	17,	68	72,	65	34,	48	72,	76
67,	72	34,	4	89,	37	90,	60	9,	23
59,	40	6,	36	81,	30	52,	38	54,	47
5,	90	29,	70	83,	71	38,	72	66,	25
44,	43	39,	54	70,	52	50,	51	95,	79
61,	81	19,	51	25,	27	51,	23	44,	26

Table 17.   Random points (x, y) in cm for sampling from rectangular surface, no side of which exceeds 1.5 metres

x	y	x	y	x	y	x	y	x	y
80,	60	55,	25	135,	135	115,	130	110,	10
80,	110	135,	35	75,	90	50,	30	10,	10
90,	90	20,	10	70,	140	40,	25	120,	135
130,	115	5,	15	80,	140	40,	80	70,	75
80,	40	50,	130	60,	110	35,	20	120,	115
145,	80	35,	40	75,	70	130,	130	140,	60
55,	135	5,	85	35,	145	60,	125	5,	105
25,	100	35,	15	65,	145	25,	135	125,	80
25,	130	50,	40	65,	40	55,	90	140,	10
35,	130	55,	30	50,	115	10,	125	90,	110
70,	85	10,	90	110,	15	120,	75	70,	70
115,	100	15,	95	130,	75	125,	105	75,	145
110,	45	120,	110	110,	115	140,	75	120,	60
85,	60	65,	75	115,	65	105,	75	75,	75
145,	50	30,	105	65,	135	90,	55	20,	145
80,	80	75,	120	15,	120	60,	75	95,	75
50,	105	100,	40	30,	5	55,	145	100,	5
65,	90	20,	70	5,	95	70,	35	40,	115
120,	30	50,	145	65,	140	115,	105	115,	95
30,	100	40,	30	110,	120	125,	120	115,	90
75,	110	30,	60	115,	15	50,	35	5,	40
115,	45	65,	120	100,	65	70,	5	100,	125
95,	115	45,	140	30,	90	60,	65	90,	30
125,	10	130,	80	120,	40	85,	80	35,	25
135,	85	40,	35	110,	50	35,	120	45,	45
15,	40	40,	5	105,	50	20,	20	90,	130
30,	75	85,	110	55,	5	115,	110	130,	35
100,	35	120,	35	10,	30	30,	10	145,	75
30,	95	140,	50	110,	100	80,	70	90,	95
35,	45	75,	95	50,	120	115,	60	35,	60
45,	95	10,	90	15,	10	55,	20	135,	15
55,	60	85,	145	100,	140	65,	95	70,	125
65,	25	105,	145	10,	110	80,	145	90,	15
95,	70	5,	100	140,	85	115,	35	30,	65
10,	100	115,	30	90,	140	145,	135	120,	95
75,	65	105,	105	35,	80	30,	25	70,	15
25,	15	110,	105	95,	95	95,	25	90,	5
55,	35	130,	65	55,	115	50,	100	5,	110
60,	80	80,	120	100,	70	40,	100	70,	65
110,	95	135,	90	70,	100	15,	130	95,	20

secondarily, because in the judgement of the investigators it appears to be typical of the population about which information is needed.   At times a decision may have to be made as to which of the two methods should be utilized since the difference in cost may be considerable.   Do we take a "chunk" and trust to our imperfect knowledge of the variability between chunks of this sort to decide how much faith we put in the estimates?   Or do we spend the money on an examination of the entire population in which we are interested so that the sampling error will be within known limits?   All that can be said on this point is that "chunk" samples may be misleading.

The stratified sampling differs from the simple random sampling in that the sampling units are in the first instance conveniently classified into several sub-populations or strata before the randomizing procedure is applied, so that the sample may be more uniformly spread over the entire population.   For instance, if we are interested in estimating the spleen rate of children, we may first divide the child population into several strata according to factors such as age-group, sex, socio-economic status, or by geographical regions.   Our purpose is to form strata in such a manner that each stratum is homogeneous internally and the different strata accordingly differ markedly from one another.   The need for stratification arises because statistics may be required separately for each stratum or that different strata may present quite different field problems which are best handled independently.   Even when these reasons do not apply, stratification is introduced to produce an increase in precision because the sample units are then more uniformly distributed over the entire population and thus various different types of population units are better represented in the sample.   If the exact size of each stratum is known a sample is taken independently from each stratum, and usually the same proportion of units are selected from each stratum.   However, when the degree of homogeneity within each stratum or the cost of surveying varies considerably from one stratum to another, theoretically it is known that in order to achieve a higher precision the sampling proportion should be varied from one stratum to another. Thus it would be more profitable to increase the sampling proportion within a stratum if it is highly variable, or if it is unusually cheap to sample.

Multi-stage sampling becomes necessary in large-scale surveys covering the population of the whole province or country for which the preparation of lists of the final sampling units such as houses or individuals for the entire population may seem impossible. In this case, as the first stage or step, a list of large-sized sampling units is prepared, such as of groups of villages lying in compact blocks comprising several thousands of persons. At the first stage a certain number of such large-sized units is selected at random. As the second stage, each of the large-sized sampling units so chosen is then considered a population by itself and sub-samples of individuals out of each unit are drawn by random sampling. The sampling being drawn in two stages, the procedure is called two-stage sampling. The process can obviously be extended to three or more stages. In some instances, quite apart from the reason of lack of a complete list of sampling units, it may be necessary, owing to administrative difficulties, to limit the number of localities to be actually surveyed. Multi-stage sampling is a solution in such cases; the entire area is subdivided into localities of a convenient size, of which several are randomly selected, and from each of the selected localities final units are then sampled. In any case the advantage of multi-stage sampling is that it gives more flexibility in the planning. The sampling error is usually higher than in the case of surveying the same number of units on the basis of simple random or stratified random sampling.

When it is considered economical and convenient to collect certain items of information from all the units of a sample (as for example data on spleen size) and other items of information from only some of these units (blood examination for instance), these latter units are so chosen as to constitute a sub-sample of the units of the original sample. This method of sampling is called multi-phase sampling. It should be noted that in multi-phase sampling, the different phases of observation relate to sample units of the same type, while in multi-stage sampling the sample units are of different types at different stages. Sometimes multi-phase sampling is used to obtain supplementary information in the second phase, to provide a more accurate estimate of information obtained in the first phase. Multi-phase sampling is therefore of use when the collection of information of a detailed nature requires much cost and labour and cannot be carried out for the entire sample.

When a number of workers are engaged in a survey it is found advantageous to arrange the drawing of two or more independent samples from each domain of study and to collect the information for each such sample in an independent manner so that each sample supplies its own independent estimate. We thus obtain what are called interpenetrating samples. It is possible to keep some of the sample units the same in two or more interpenetrating networks of samples so that information for such sample units is independently collected twice or more. It is then possible to make detailed comparisons between two or more sets of observations. Interpenetrating samples are thus found useful to secure information on non-sampling errors such as differences arising from differential bias of the investigator, different methods of eliciting the information, etc. The interpenetrating network therefore provides a means of control or appraisal of the quality of the information collected.

Sometimes, instead of drawing a random sample from serially numbered units we may carry out "systematic sampling" by selecting every fifth or tenth, etc. unit on the list. For this purpose, if we are to select let us say every kth unit, we first draw a random number "r" lying between one and "k", so that the first unit randomly chosen in the sample from the list is the rth unit. Thereafter we select the $(r + k)$th, the $(r + 2k)$th and so on until the list is finished. Thus, if a part of the population contains 34 units to be sampled at 20%, or 1 in 5, we select a random number between 1 and 5, say 2. The sample consists of the units with the numbers 2, 7, 12, 17, 22, 27 and 32. This type of sample, called the systematic sample, is easier to select than a simple random sample, particularly if the drawing is to be done by the field staff. It is likely to be more accurate than a simple random sample if there is a trend in the measurement which follows the order of numbering. All the same, the use of this technique may be risky. For instance, if it happens in sampling houses that every fifth house is situated at the corner of a street the sample selected by the above technique may either contain corner houses only or exclude them altogether. Thus the validity of the sample will be vitiated. Another defect of this method is that the exact formula is not available for estimating the sampling error. In general practice the sampling error of a systematic sample is approximately estimated by applying the formula for the random sampling as a convenient substitute.

2.20.4   The question of non-response

In sampling human populations the problem invariably arises of difficulty in contacting, examining or interviewing people.   Some are unable to or unwilling to be examined and this is particularly so in surveys where the data desired involve some inconvenience to the person such as the drawing of blood for the detection of infection.   Any sizable percentage of non-response would make the results obviously open to question.   Sometimes non-response is allowed for by substituting other individuals for those who were hard to find or non-cooperative.   But substitutes rarely solve the problem.   They merely increase the size of the sample in that section of the population which is amenable to our survey.   If the non-response is due to difficulty in contacting the respondent or to unwillingness to co-operate, one method is to concentrate on a random sub-sample chosen out of the non-responding cases and to make every effort possible to obtain the data from individuals falling in this sub-sample so that some information may be obtained with respect to the non-respondent group in the population.

The problem of non-response assumes considerable importance when information is sought by means of questionnaires and then replies of volunteers are analysed. The response depends upon the auspices of the study, the length of the questionnaire, the format of the questionnaire, and many other factors.   However, it is not so well known that the characteristics of those who do not respond may differ widely from those who do.   Consequently reliance upon statistical results based on tabulation of questionnaires from those who took the trouble to reply may lead to false conclusions.   It is not justifiable to assume that those who have replied form a representative sample of those to whom a questionnaire was sent.   How to overcome this bias and at the same time make use of the undoubted economies which can often be achieved by the questionnaire is a matter on which an experienced statistician's advice should be sought.

2.20.5   Pilot survey

It is recommended that a pilot survey be first carried out in order to obtain information which will facilitate the planning and executing of the main survey. The main purposes of a pilot survey are:

(1)   to examine survey techniques to be used - such as adequacy of various definitions, design of the questionnaire, interviewing method, etc.;

(2)   to obtain necessary data on the variability existing in sampling units in order to provide some rough basis for stratification and estimation of the sampling error;

(3)   to obtain data on the amount of labour and money required to carry out the main survey;

(4)   to give the staff an opportunity to get accustomed to the various other problems met with in executing the main survey.

The pilot survey should preferably provide information in such a manner that it shall be possible to incorporate it into the body of the information provided later by the main survey.   In other words we will be conducting a survey in two instalments, namely (i) the pilot survey, and (ii) the main survey, the method and scope of sampling for the latter being provided by the pilot survey.

2.20.6   Bias

If, either due to the subjective or personal error of the investigator, or the faulty technique of randomization, there is a consistent over-estimation or under-estimation of the average value, the sample estimate is said to be biased.   Bias can also be introduced through forgetfulness on the part of the informants or through the refusal of individuals to supply accurate information or through the use of unreliable diagnostic techniques.   Such bias cannot be reduced or eliminated by increasing the number of observations, but only by the adoption of sound sampling and survey techniques.

2.20.7 Recommendations of the United Nations Sub-Commission on Statistical Sampling

The United Nations Sub-Commission on Statistical Sampling has set out certain recommendations for the preparation of reports on sampling surveys and to standardize technical terminology with a view to ensuring clarity, comprehensiveness and international comparability in the reports that deal with the aims, methods used and accuracy obtained in sampling surveys. A full discussion of these recommendations is contained in the United Nations (1950) document "The preparation of sampling survey reports". The following summary of the principal recommendations of the Sub-Commission is reproduced from United Nations Statistical Office Paper (United Nations, 1955) on statistical sampling.

(a) A general description of any survey should be given with regard to the scope and purposes of the survey, the material covered, nature of the information collected, method of collecting the data, sampling method, accuracy, cost, and an assessment of the extent to which the purposes of the survey were fulfilled, etc.

(b) A description of the design of the survey should clearly specify the domain of study, the frame[1] used for selecting the sample, the distinction between elementary observation units and sample units; and should provide full information on schemes of stratification, if any, sampling fractions within strata, stages and phases of sampling and provision of any means of controlling or appraising the quality of the data collected, as for example the adoption of interpenetrating or replicated sampling. The description of the design should conform as far as possible to current established terminology.

(c) The method used in the selection of the sample units should be described.

(d) An account should be given of the personnel employed and the equipment used.

---

[1] The frame consists of previously available descriptions of the material in the form of maps, lists, directories, etc. from which sample units may be constructed and a set of units selected.

(e)   The statistical methods followed in the compilation of the final summary tables and the computational procedure used should be described.

(f)   Information should be given on the cost of the survey, classified so far as possible under the various headings listed in the report.

(g)   Information concerning the accuracy of the survey as indicated by the random sampling errors deducible from the survey, non-sampling errors, accuracy and adequacy of the frame, comparison with other sources of information, etc. should be included.

2.21   Estimation of LD_{50} or LC_{50} - Probit Analysis

2.21.1   Terminology used

In order to ascertain whether mosquitos in an area are likely to develop resistance following insecticide spraying, it is necessary, in the first instance, to measure what their degree of susceptibility is before the commencement of insecticide spraying operations in that area.   This base-line information, if recorded in numerical terms, should enable us to make comparisons with similar figures at later periods.   Such numerical assessment should also be made when comparing the degree of susceptibility of mosquitos of the same or different species in different places.   A numerical index of the degree of susceptibility is therefore needed.

It is customary for this purpose to estimate experimentally for any batch of insects the concentration of the insecticide that would kill half the number of mosquitos (50%) exposed to the insecticide.   It is of course understood that the experimental conditions and the technique of measuring such a concentration level should be the standard ones, otherwise variation in concentration values would arise not only from possible changes in the degree of susceptibility of mosquitos but also from differences in experimental techniques and the conditions in respect of temperature, humidity, etc. under which the estimation is made.   The WHO Expert Committee on Malaria (WHO, 1954) recommended the Busvine & Nash method as the standard technique for the purpose of ensuring uniformity.   The techniques used should be based on these principles.   According to this method mosquitos are exposed in specimen tubes lined with filter paper impregnated with the insecticide for a fixed period of one hour at 27°C temperature.   The degree of impregnation of the filter paper differs from tube to tube, for example, in the case of DDT, the concentrations used are 4%, 2%, 1% and 0.5%

After such exposure the mosquitos are transferred to cages kept at 27°C and mortality counts are made after 24 hours. The need for exposing mosquitos to varying concentrations of the insecticide all at the same time arises from the fact that in the experiment we expect the higher concentration to kill more than 50% of mosquitos and the least concentration to kill fewer than 50%, so that the concentration expected to kill 50% would lie within this range. Table 18 shows the mortality of A. sacharovi 24 hours after exposure to various concentrations of DDT in a test carried out in Ghantargholou, Iran, in September 1956 (de Zulueta's unpublished data). The last column of this table shows mortality rates ranging between 12.9% and 100.0% corresponding to the various concentrations of the insecticide.

Table 18. Mortality of A. sacharovi exposed to various concentrations of DDT, Ghantargholou, Iran September 1956

DDT concentration in %	Total number of mosquitos tested	Number of mosquitos dead in 24 hours	Mortality rate (%)
0.5	31	4	12.9
1.0	34	17	50.0
2.0	36	30	83.3
4.0	27	27	100.0
Control	38	2	5.3

As stated already, we need to summarize the result of this experiment by a single numerical index and accordingly we proceed to calculate the concentration that should have, under the same experimental conditions, resulted in a 50% kill. In statistical terminology this concentration level is called the "median lethal dose" and is expressed by the symbol LD_{50} (lethal dose 50). It is not abbreviated to MLD as this abbreviation is likely to be misinterpreted to mean also the minimum lethal dose, i.e. the concentration at which the mortality of mosquitos begins to rise above the natural level. The term LC_{50} is also used; the letter C signifying concentration, i.e. the concentration of the insecticide to produce 50% kill.

In accordance with this notation, the level of the insecticide concentration at which mortality rates of 10%, 20%, ..., 90%, etc. are expected to occur would be denoted by the symbols LD_{10}, LD_{20}, ..., LD_{90}, etc. respectively, or LC_{10}, LC_{20}, ... LC_{90}, etc. The reason why LD_{50} is used in preference to LDs at other percentage levels of mortality is that usually the value of LD_{50} is obtainable with a higher degree of precision than the other values. In other words the experimental error associated with LD_{50} is generally of a lower order than that accompanying other LD values.

2.21.2 Adjustment for natural mortality

The Busvine & Nash method also recommends that the test should provide for controls, i.e. the mosquitos should also be exposed to paper treated with an insecticide-free volatile solvent mixture. The mortality recorded among mosquitos so exposed (control mortality) is then due merely to natural causes. Each of the mortality percentages observed among mosquitos exposed to the insecticide should first be adjusted to allow for natural mortality. The formula, called Abbot's formula, is used to obtain adjusted mortality percentages which are used to calculate LD_{50}. The recorded percentage mortality of mosquitos at each concentration is separately adjusted by the formula:

$$\text{Adjusted mortality percentage} = \frac{\text{Actual mortality percentage} - \text{Control mortality percentage}}{100 - \text{Control mortality percentage}} \times 100$$

Example:

Suppose the observed mortality was 12.9% and the mortality for the control group was 5.3%, then the adjusted mortality percentage is equal to:

$$\frac{12.9 - 5.3}{100 - 5.3} \times 100 = \frac{7.6}{94.7} \times 100 = 8.0\%$$

Owing to chance variation it may sometimes happen that the control mortality percentage is higher than the lowest figure of mortality percentage observed among mosquitos exposed to the insecticide. In that case, the lowest figure recorded in the experiment may be used for control mortality by which to adjust the other values of mortality percentages.

In Table 19 are given the values of adjusted mortality (column 3) for the susceptibility data of A. sacharovi shown in Table 18.

Table 19.   Observed and adjusted mortality of A. sacharovi
data from Iran, September 1956

DDT concentration in %	Observed mortality (%)	Adjusted mortality (%)
0.5	12.9	8.0
1.0	50.0	47.2
2.0	83.3	82.4
4.0	100.0	100.0
Control	5.3	

2.21.3   Graphical methods of estimating LD$_{50}$

One of the simplest methods of estimating LD$_{50}$ could be to plot the observed percentage mortality (corrected for natural mortality) as in Fig. 20.   Concentration level is marked along the horizontal axis and the corresponding percentage mortality along the vertical axis.   Such mortality percentages are known to fall along a flattened "S" shaped curve as has been drawn freehand in the figure, to pass as closely as possible to all the plotted points.   In order to read the value of LD$_{50}$ from this curve, a horizontal line is drawn from the 50% mortality level to cut the "S" shaped curve at point "P".   From point "P" a vertical line is drawn to cut the horizontal axis at "M".   The concentration marked by point "M" is the concentration that would be expected to produce a 50% kill, which is the value of LD$_{50}$ estimated graphically.

Even though it may seem easy to draw a freehand "S" shaped curve, different individuals and especially inexperienced ones are likely to draw curves which might vary from person to person, and thus slightly different estimates of the value of LD$_{50}$ would be obtained from the same data by different workers.

Another approximate method which may, to some extent, eliminate the personal bias of the individual is to use a specially designed graph sheet, called the "probit log" paper. Both the horizontal and vertical axes in this sheet are specially marked at unequal intervals in such a manner that if the mortality conforms to a certain theoretical model, then the points of observed mortality should fall along a straight line. Actually, the horizontal axis is marked according to the logarithmic scale and the vertical axis according to what is called the "probit" scale. (The term "probit" is explained in a later paragraph.) Of course to facilitate the plotting of the points, the scales bear actual figures of insecticide concentration and the recorded figures of corresponding percentage mortality (see Fig. 21). The observed data can thus be directly plotted on such a probit log sheet - each pair of observations again corresponding to a point. When using this probit log sheet, instead of attempting to draw freehand an "S" shaped curve we hold a ruler in such a manner that a straight line would seem to the eye to pass as near as possible to all the points. In drawing such a line it is necessary to bear in mind that greater importance is to be attached to those mortality levels at which a relatively larger number of mosquitos was used. It is known from statistical theory that when an equal number of mosquitos are tested at each level, the points around the mortality level of 50% are of greater importance than those corresponding to extreme mortality values such as those near 0% or 100%. As a matter of fact, points corresponding to mortalities of exactly 0% and 100% provide little information for the estimation of LD_{50}. In fitting a straight line to the points by the eye we may ignore points corresponding to the mortality percentages of 0% and 100% as well as the values close to these two percentages. A straight-line relationship thus observed is not only more convenient for the purpose of graphically estimating LD_{50} but is also useful for the subsequent numerical calculation of the more precise estimate of LD_{50} by methods referred to in a later paragraph. A straight line fitted by the eye to the points on a probit log paper provides a first approximation to what is called the "probit regression line".

Fig. 20.   Relationship between concentration of DDT and percentage
mortality of <u>A. sacharovi</u> (Dr de Zulueta's data)

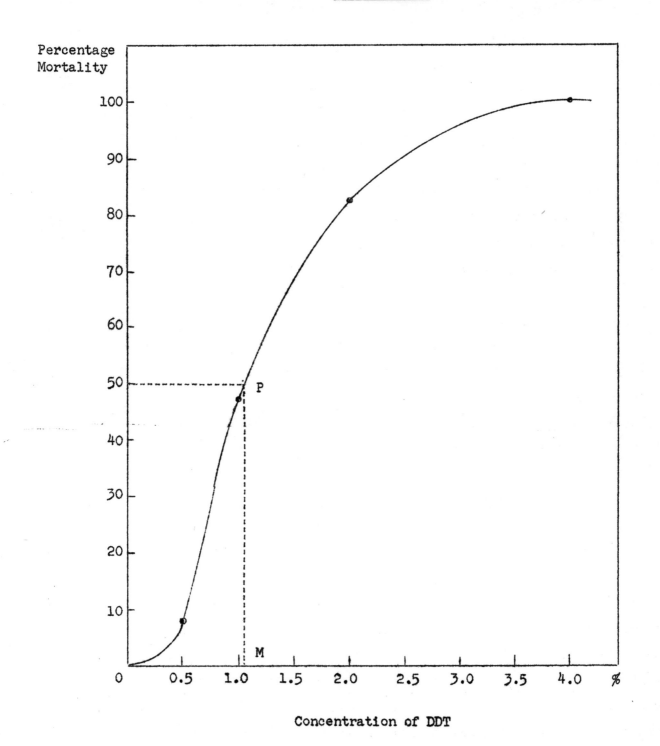

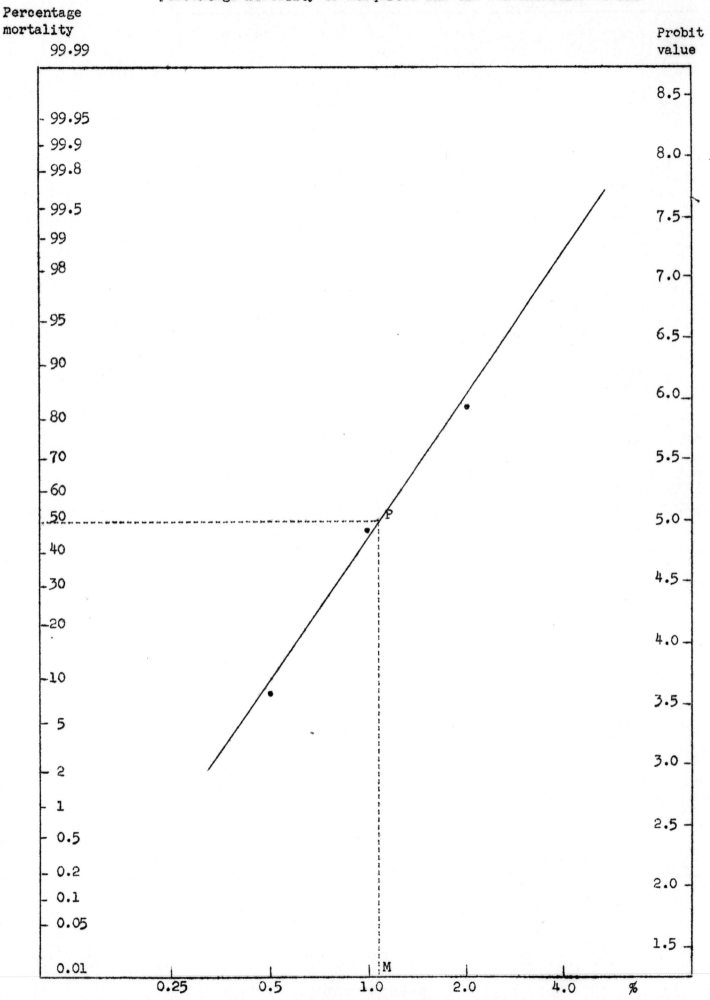

Fig. 21.   Probit log paper showing the straight-line relationship between percentage mortality of mosquitos and the concentration of DDT

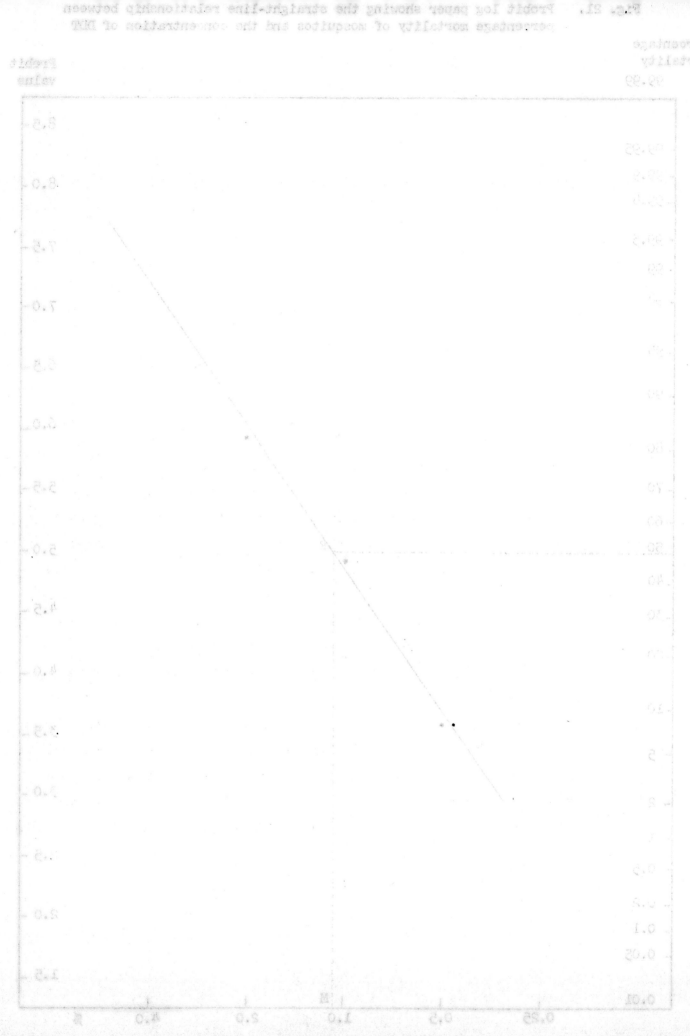

The graphical method of estimating LD_{50} from this straight line then consists
in reading from the line the concentration level corresponding to 50% mortality.
More specifically we draw a horizontal line through the 50% mortality level to cut
the probit regression line at the point "P".   A vertical line is then drawn through
the point P to cut the horizontal axis at M.   The point M then marks the LD_{50}, the
value of which can be read from the scale (see Fig. 21).   For instance, the figure
shows that the data presented in Table 19 (first and third columns) give 1.1% as
the graphical value of LD_{50}.

2.21.4   Litchfield & Wilcoxon's short-cut method

2.21.4.1   Estimation of LD_{50}

The graphical estimate of LD_{50} obtained above is needed for deriving more
refined estimates by computational procedures explained in later paragraphs.
But such computational procedures are difficult and laborious, so much so that
some workers may be deterred from using them.   With the aim of introducing ease
of computation without undue sacrifice of efficiency and accuracy a convenient
scheme has been devised by Litchfield & Wilcoxon (1949).   They use the probit log
paper and begin by fitting a line by the eye as has been explained above.   But in
the first instance any 0% and 100% values are disregarded.   The expected values
of mortality percentage are then read from the line corresponding to those dose
levels, which in the experiment had provided 0% or 100% values.   Corresponding
to these expected values the corrected percentage values are read from the table
below (Table 20).   The corrected expected values are now plotted on the same chart.
Taking these additional points also into account a new line is fitted by the eye.
If the new line is found to differ much from the previously fitted line, then new
expected values are read from the second line, and recorrected from Table 20 and
again plotted.   When the line appears to fit satisfactorily, the value corresponding
to 50% is read graphically as LD_{50}.

Example:

In applying the above method to the data shown in Table 19 we first plot points on probit log paper corresponding to the concentration levels of 0.5%, 1% and 2%, i.e. cases in which mortality rates were neither 0% nor 100% (Fig. 22). A tentative line AA' is drawn to pass as near as possible to the three points plotted. From this line the expected percentage mortality value corresponding to the dose 4% is read graphically as 98.6%. By referring to Table 20[1] below, the value of corrected mortality corresponding to the expected value of 98.6% is found to be 99.5% by interpolation. This corrected mortality value is also now plotted on the same chart and a new line BB' is drawn by taking all the four points into consideration. The graphical value corresponding to the dose of 4% concentration is now 99% and from Table 20 the corresponding corrected value is found to be 99.7% - a close enough figure. However, as is explained in the next section we test whether the second line has provided a satisfactory fit. If the fit were found to be unsatisfactory we would repeat the procedure outlined above. We have to keep in mind that it is the concentration value corresponding to 50% mortality in which we are interested and the effect of such improved fits of the line may not produce much difference in LD_{50} value. The value of LD_{50} as read from the graph (line BB') is 1.07%.

Table 20.   Corrected values of 0% or 100% effect corresponding to expected values[1]

Expected	0	1	2	3	4	5	6	7	8	9
0	–	0.3	0.7	1.0	1.3	1.6	2.0	2.3	2.6	2.9
10	3.2	3.5	3.8	4.1	4.4	4.7	4.9	5.2	5.5	5.7
20	6.0	6.2	6.5	6.7	7.0	7.2	7.4	7.6	7.8	8.1
30	8.3	8.4	8.6	8.8	9.0	9.2	9.3	9.4	9.6	9.8
40	9.9	10.0	10.1	10.2	10.3	10.3	10.4	10.4	10.4	10.5
50	–	89.5	89.6	89.6	89.6	89.7	89.7	89.8	89.9	90.0
60	90.1	90.2	90.4	90.5	90.7	90.8	91.0	91.2	91.4	91.6
70	91.7	91.9	92.2	92.4	92.6	92.8	93.0	93.3	93.5	93.8
80	94.0	94.3	94.5	94.8	95.1	95.3	95.6	95.9	96.2	96.5
90	96.8	97.1	97.4	97.7	98.0	98.4	98.7	99.0	99.3	99.7

---

[1] The column headings 0 to 9 represent the units place while the first column represents the tens place. Thus to read the corrected value corresponding to expected value of 98% refer to the table at the row marked 90 and the column marked 8 and read the corrected figure as 99.3.

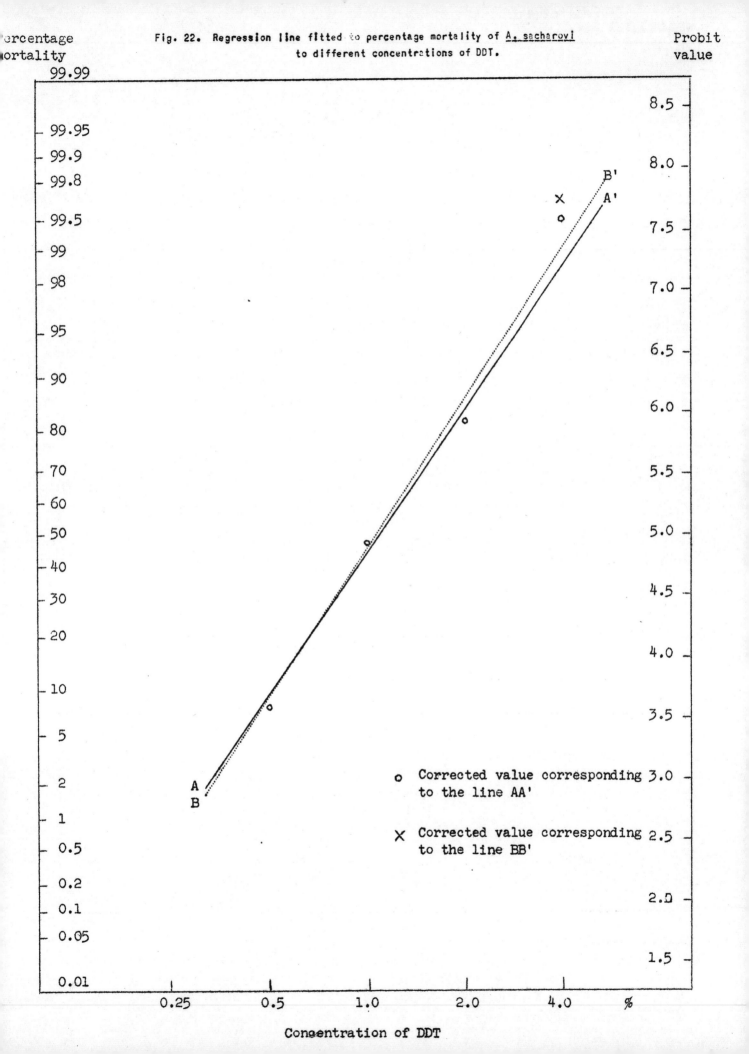

Fig. 22. Regression line fitted to percentage mortality of _A. sacharovi_ to different concentrations of DDT.

Fig. 85. Regression line (Bliss) percentage mortality of A. stephensi to different concentrations of DDT.

2.21.4.2 <u>Goodness of fit of probit regression line</u>

By a simple computation the goodness of fit of the probit regression line to the data may be assessed numerically. For this purpose first we read from the probit log diagram the difference between the observed and the expected mortality percentage values at each dose level. The following quantity d is then computed for each concentration level:

$$d = \frac{(\text{Observed} - \text{expected per cent. mortality})^2}{(\text{Expected per cent. mortality}) \times (100 - \text{expected per cent. mortality})}$$

Values for different concentration levels are then added and the sum multiplied by the average number of mosquitos per dose.

$$X^2 = (\text{Total of d}) \times (\text{average number of mosquitos per does})$$

This quantity X^2 is a measure of the goodness of fit of the probit regression line to the points; the smaller the value the better relatively is the fit. This value X^2 should be compared with the critical X^2 value tabulated in Appendix D. The corresponding degrees of freedom are the number of concentration levels minus 2. In case the computed value of X^2 is found to exceed the corresponding critical value the indication is that the line is not a satisfactory fit to the observed data. A new regression line should then be fitted by the eye to reduce the larger values of d and the value of X^2 computed again. This process is repeated until the X^2 value is reduced below the critical value.

In some instances the computed value of X^2 cannot possibly be reduced below the permissible value by a choice of the line. In such cases the cause of the excessive value of the computed X^2 lies in the heterogeneity of the original data. The line giving the smallest X^2 value is to be chosen as the regression line and the value of LD_{50} is read from this line as usual. However, the computation of the upper and lower confidence limits (see next section) need modifying to allow for heterogeneity of the data.

Litchfield & Wilcoxon have provided monograms by means of which the compilation of X^2 can be facilitated by obtaining the values of d at a glance.

Example:

In the example given in the previous paragraph the value of X^2 is computed as shown in Table 21.

Table 21. Calculating the value of X^2 for the fitted probit
regression line

Concentration of DDT	Observed mortality *	Expected mortality	$\dfrac{[(2)-(3)]^2}{(3)\times[100-(3)]}$
(1)	(2)	(3)	(4)
0.5	8.0	9.0	0.0012
1.0	47.2	45.0	0.0020
2.0	82.4	86.2	0.0121
4.0	99.7	99.0**	0.0049
Total			0.0202

* Observed mortality adjustment for natural mortality.

** For the concentration level which experimentally gave 0% or 100% mortality, the corrected mortality value is to be used in the computation of X^2.

Total number of mosquitos tested at four concentration levels

$= 31 + 34 + 36 + 27 = 128$

$\therefore X^2 = 0.0202 \times \dfrac{128}{4} = 0.646$

The critical value of X^2 corresponding to two degrees of freedom (4 levels - 2) is 5.99 at 5% probability level. The computed value is less than the critical value and therefore the goodness of fit of the regression line is within the permissible limit.

2.21.4.3   Confidence limits of LD_{50}

The authors provide a simple method of estimating the upper and lower confidence limits within which the LD_{50} is expected to lie with 95% (or 99%) probability.

For this purpose the probit regression line is used also to read graphically the dose values corresponding to LD_{16} and LD_{84}.   For these values, a quantity S is calculated by means of the following formula:

$$S = \frac{LD_{84}/LD_{50} + LD_{50}/LD_{16}}{2}$$

From the original data we work out the total number of mosquitos tested at all those dose levels which lie between LD_{16} and LD_{84} and denote the total number by N. Next we substitute the values of S and N in the following formula to find the value of "f" - the factor by which LD_{50} should be multiplied and divided to obtain respectively the upper and lower values of confidence limits at 95%:

$$\text{Log } f_{95} = \frac{2.77}{\sqrt{N}} \log S$$

If the confidence limits are required at 99% probability level the formula to be used for "f" is:

$$\log f_{99} = \frac{3.641}{\sqrt{N}} \log S$$

Litchfield & Wilcoxon provide nomograms by means of which the confidence limits can be estimated without recourse to logarithms.

When heterogeneity exists in the original data (see section 2.21.4.2) the formula to be used is:

$$\log f = 1.41 \ t \sqrt{\frac{\chi^2}{n \ N}} \ ,$$

where t is the critical value of the t-distribution shown in Appendix E, corresponding to the degrees of freedom n, i.e. the number of concentration levels minus 2, and N is the number of mosquitos tested at those dose levels which lie between LD_{16} and LD_{84}.

Example:

In the example given above the values of LD_{16} and LD_{84} are read from the line BB' of Fig. 22 as follows:

$$LD_{16} = 0.61\% , \quad LD_{84} = 1.9\%$$

$$LD_{50} = 1.07\%$$

By using these values we obtain:

$$S = \frac{LD_{84}/LD_{50} + LD_{50}/LD_{16}}{2} = \frac{1.9/1.07 + 1.07/0.61}{2} = 1.76$$

$$\log S = 0.2455$$

The number of mosquitos tested at concentration levels between LD_{16} and LD_{84} is 34.

$$\therefore N = 34 , \quad \sqrt{N} = 5.83$$

$$\log f_{95} = \frac{2.77}{\sqrt{N}} \log S = \frac{2.77}{5.83} \times 0.2455 = 0.1166$$

$$f_{95} = 1.31$$

The 95% confidence limits are therefore:

$$1.07\% \times 1.31 = 1.40\% \quad \text{and}$$
$$1.07\% = 1.31 = 0.82\%$$

2.21.5 Numerical method of estimating LD_{50}

For the purpose of obtaining a numerical estimate of LD_{50} we first work out the logarithms of the concentration value of the insecticide (see Appendix A). The working out of logarithmic values is facilitated if each percentage concentration value is multiplied by a convenient figure, say 10 or 100, so that all the concentrations used in the test are transformed to figures greater than 1.

Each recorded mortality percentage is converted to what is called the probit value. In practice all that is required is to read from ready-reckoning tables the probit value set out against each mortality percentage. Table 22 is given in a condensed form merely to show the correspondence in the values read out. At the bottom of this table are also given the values for the percentage mortality recorded in our numerical example.

Table 22. Probit values corresponding to mortality percentage figures

Observed percentage mortality	Probit value
1	2.67
2	2.95
3	3.12
4	3.25
5	3.36
10	3.72
15	3.96
20	4.16
25	4.33
30	4.48
35	4.61
40	4.75
45	4.87
50	5.00
55	5.13
60	5.25
65	5.39
70	5.52
75	5.67
80	5.84
85	6.04
90	6.28
95	6.64
96	6.75
97	6.88
98	7.05
99	7.33
8.0	3.59
47.2	4.93
82.4	5.93

In actual practice it will be necessary of course to use a more detailed table giving probit values corresponding to percentage mortalities at intervals of 0.1%. Such a table is provided by Fisher & Yates (1953) (Table IX, pages 60-62) and should be available for the numerical estimation of LD_{50}. The purpose of the explanation given in the following paragraphs is merely to indicate the computational procedures involved in this work.

From the above table we can see that the probit value corresponding to 50% mortality is exactly 5.0. The probit value increases with increasing percentage mortality so that for 95% mortality the probit value is 6.64. The probit values corresponding to 0% and 100% mortality are minus infinity and plus infinity respectively, which of course cannot be plotted on the graph.

The figures given in Table 19 are shown below (Table 23) converted to logarithmic values of the insecticide concentration and the probit value of mortality as read out from ready-made tables, e.g. either from Finney (1952), pages 264-267 or from Table IX of Fisher & Yates (1953).

Table 23.   Probit value of mortality and logarithmic value
of concentration

Insecticide concentration		Mortality	
Percentage values x 10	Logarithm of concentration	Percentage[*]	Probit value
5	0.699	8.0	3.59
10	1.000	47.2	4.93
20	1.301	82.4	5.93
40	1.602	100.0	oo

[*] Corrected for control mortality.

The reason why we have converted the observed mortality percentage to the probit scale and the concentration value of insecticide to the logarithmic scale is that if we now plot the probit values against logarithmic concentration values the points are expected to fall along a straight line. Of course, if the probit log sheet is used we can just as well plot the untransformed data, as in Fig. 21, but the conversion of these values as carried out in the above table is necessary for the subsequent numerical calculation of LD_{50}. The formula for calculating LD_{50} differs when there is no natural mortality from the case where mortality among the controls is also recorded.

2.21.5.1 Estimating LD_{50} when there is no natural mortality

In this paragraph the procedure applicable to a case in which there is no natural mortality is explained. As an example, however, the same data are taken as are quoted in previous paragraphs, which included a control group with the mortality of 5.3%. These data are analysed by regarding the values of adjusted mortality (by Abbott's formula) as if they were actually observed mortality values and as if there were no natural mortality. This approximation is permissible when the control mortality is small or it is based on a large number of observations. The precise method allowing for the natural mortality is explained in the next paragraph, where this example is re-analysed by the more appropriate method.

Having plotted the points we first draw a probit regression line freehand as explained in section 2.21.3 (Fig. 21). The expected value of the probit (denoted by the letter Y) corresponding to each logarithmic concentration is read out from the line. For instance, corresponding to the logarithmic concentration value of 0.699 (concentration of 0.5%), the graph shows that the expected probit value of Y is 3.7. In the same manner the probit regression line gives the expected probit value of 4.9, corresponding to logarithmic concentration of 1.000 (concentration of 1%). In so far as these values of expected probit would vary according to variations in the fitting of the probit regression line by the eye, they are to be considered only as first approximations. These figures are shown in column 4 of Table 24.

Table 24. <u>Estimation of LD$_{50}$ when there is no natural mortality</u>

Logarithmic concentration	Number of mosquitos tested	Percentage mortality	Expected probit (graphical)	Weight	Working probit
x	n	p	Y	w	·y
(1)	(2)	(3)	(4)	(5)	(6)·
0.699	31	8.0	3.7	10.4	3.60
1.000	34	47.2	4.9	21.6	4.93
1.301	36	82.4	6.0	15.8	5.93
1.602	27	100.0	7.2	2.5	7.59

The expected probit values (Y) as read from the line are next converted into what
are called the "working probit values" (y) by means of the following formula:

$$y = y_o + kp$$

In this formula, p corresponds to the observed percentage mortality (column 3 of
Table 24).   The values of y_o and k corresponding to each graphically obtained
probit value (Y) are read from Fisher & Yates (1953) (Table XI)[1] and substituted
in this equation.   A condensed form of the table is given below to illustrate its
use (Table 25).   At the bottom of this table the values for those figures which
appear in the numerical example are also shown.   As an example we may calculate
the working probit y corresponding to the percentage mortality 8.0.   The expected
probit Y corresponding to this percentage mortality is 3.7 (see Table 24).   By
referring to Table 25 we find that corresponding to the Y value of 3.7, y_o is 3.1351
and k is 0.058354.   Therefore the working probit y = 3.1351 + 0.058354 x 8.0 = 3.602.
Column (6) of Table 24 shows the values of y for each level of concentration.

---

[1] In these tables y_o is denoted as Y - P/Z and a symbol 1/Z is used instead of k.
In applying their tables the mortality values should be used in fractions and not in
percentages.

Table 25.   Values of constants y_0 and k for computation
of the working probit

Y	y_0	k
2.0	1.6954	2.256395
2.5	2.1457	0.570506
3.0	2.5786	0.185216
3.5	2.9842	0.077210
4.0	3.3443	0.041327
4.5	3.6236	0.028404
5.0	3.7467	0.025066
5.5	3.5360	0.028404
6.0	2.5230	0.041327
6.5	-0.7051	0.077210
7.0	-11.1002	0.185216
7.5	-49.1963	0.570506
8.0	-217.3349	2.256395
3.7	3.1351	0.058354
4.9	3.7407	0.025192
6.0	2.5230	0.041327
7.2	-20.5973	0.281892

As mentioned earlier, we have to attach greater or lesser importance to each percentage mortality depending on the number of mosquitos that were used in the test and also depending on whether the observed percentage mortality is near about the 50% level or is further removed from it.   The weight to be thus attached to each probit value is provided by what is called the "weighting coefficient" which can be read from a ready-reckoning table published by Fisher & Yates (1953), Table XI. As an illustration, the values of the weighting coefficient are shown in Table 26 for selected probit values.

Table 26.   Weighting coefficients corresponding to various
expected probit values

Y	Weighting coefficients
2.0	.01457
2.5	.04979
3.0	.13112
3.5	.26907
4.0	.43863
4.5	.58099
5.0	.63662
5.5	.58099
6.0	.43863
6.5	.26907
7.0	.13112
7.5	.04979
8.0	.01457
3.7	.33589
4.9	.63431
6.0	.43863
7.2	.09179

The weighting coefficient is further multiplied by the corresponding number of mosquitos tested.   Thus, for the first concentration level in our numerical example, the weighting coefficient as read from Table 26 corresponding to the expected value (Y) of 3.7 is 0.33589.   Therefore the weight to be assigned to this concentration is $w = 31 \times 0.33589 = 10.4$.   Column 5 of Table 24 shows the values of the weight (w) for all the expected probit Y values of the test.   With the help of the values of x, y and w as explained by various column headings in Table 24, we next prepare the following Table 27 in which the headings show the multiplications to be carried out. The total of each column is shown in the last row.

Table 27. Computational procedure for estimating LD_{50}

x	y	w	wx	wx^2	wy	wxy
(1)	(2)	(3)	(4)	(5)	(6)	(7)
0.699	3.60	10.4	7.27	5.08	37.44	26.17
1.000	4.93	21.6	21.60	21.60	106.49	106.49
1.301	5.93	15.8	20.56	26.75	93.69	121.90
1.602	7.59	2.5	4.01	6.42	18.98	30.40
Total		50.3	53.44	59.85	256.60	284.96

The values of two constants, a and b, required in a later formula are then calculated by substituting the values from Table 27 in the following formula:

$$b = \frac{S(w)\,S(wxy) - S(wx)\,S(wy)}{S(w)\,S(wx^2) - [S(wx)]^2} = \frac{50.3 \times 284.96 - 53.44 \times 256.60}{50.3 \times 59.85 - (53.44)^2} = 4.01$$

$$a = \frac{S(wy)}{Sw} - b\frac{S(wx)}{Sw} = \frac{256.60}{50.3} - 4.01 \times \frac{53.44}{50.3} = 0.841$$

By using the formula $Y' = a + bx$, we calculate new probit values Y' corresponding to each value of logarithm of concentration (x) as shown below:

x	Y'	Y
0.699	3.64	3.7
1.000	4.85	4.9
1.301	6.06	6.0
1.602	7.27	7.2

The probit values Y' are compared with the expected probit value Y obtained earlier graphically (column 4 of Table 24). It will be seen that both values show no appreciable differences. If that is so, the value of logarithm LD_{50} is obtained by the following formula:

$$\text{Log LD}_{50} = \frac{5 - a}{b}$$

In the present example, $\text{Log LD}_{50} = \dfrac{5 - 0.841}{4.01} = 1.037$

The antilog of the above figure is 10.9 which is the value of LD_{50}. In order to obtain the LD_{50} in terms of percentage concentration, this value should be divided by 10, which provides us with the value of 1.09%.

In the above computation we have found that the value of Y' and Y did not appreciably differ and therefore we could proceed to calculate the LD_{50}. If the graphical estimate has been made carefully, it usually happens that Y and Y' are similar in magnitude. In case the difference is appreciable then a second series of estimates of expected probits should be made by treating the Y' values as if they were the values obtained from graphical method. In that case, a second cycle of numerical calculations according to steps outlined above, should be followed to obtain a new series of probit values to resemble those of Y'.

This procedure of revising the values more than once in order to ensure that the last two estimates do not differ appreciably from each other is called the process of "iteration".

2.21.5.2 Computation of LD_{50} by allowing for natural mortality

When the figure of percentage mortality for the control group is available, the mortality percentages observed in the test groups should each be adjusted first by applying Abbott's formula as stated in paragraph 2.21.2. The subsequent procedure to obtain the value of the LD_{50} is essentially similar to the one discussed in the preceding paragraph for cases where no natural mortality is involved. However, some additional computation is involved, owing to the fact that the natural mortality as estimated from the mortality experience of the control group is also subject to an experimental error. The procedure consists in starting with a provisional value of the natural mortality and a provisional probit regression line.

These provisional estimates are then revised.   When the revised values do not differ materially from the provisional ones, the revised values are used in the estimation of LD_{50}.   If they do, then the revised values are regarded as the first approximation and a second cycle of computation is undertaken to revise them again.   The necessary steps for the revision of the provisional probit values or for the revision of the calculated probit values are explained below with the help of our numerical example.

We have already noted that in Dr de Zulueta's experiment a control group consisting of 38 mosquitos was provided, out of which 2 mosquitos died after 24 hours (Table 18).   The mortality from natural causes or control mortality then is:

$$\frac{2}{38} \times 100 \text{ or } 5.3\%$$

As stated already, the control mortality of 5.3% estimated from only a limited number of mosquitos is itself associated with error.   For the sake of simplicity we may start with a provisional value for the natural mortality of 5%.   The first step to be taken then is to adjust the observed mortality of the test group by Abbott's formula (see paragraph 2.21.2) and thereby obtain the corresponding probit value of each adjusted mortality from Fisher & Yates, Table IX.   Thus we get the figures in Table 28.

Table 28.   Mortality of A. sacharovi exposed to various concentrations of DDT. Ghantargholou, Iran, September 1956 (Dr de Zulueta's data)

Concentration of DDT (x 10)	Logarithm of concentration x	Number of mosquitos tested n	Number of mosquitos dead r	Observed percentage mortality	Adjusted percentage mortality p (natural mortality $K_0 = 5\%$)	Probit value of p
(1)	(2)	(3)	(4)	(5)	(6)	(7)
5	0.699	31	4	12.9	8.3	3.61
10	1.000	34	17	50.0	47.4	4.93
20	1.301	36	30	83.3	82.4	5.93
40	1.602	27	27	100.0	100.0	oo
Control group		38	2	5.263		

The probit values thus obtained (column 7 of Table 28) are then plotted against the logarithmic values of concentration and a provisional probit regression line is drawn so that the line will pass as near to all the points as possible, by taking into account the relative weight of the points (see paragraph 2.21.3).   Figure 23 shows such a provisional regression line for our example.

The "expected probit value" (denoted by Y) is next read from the regression line corresponding to each logarithmic concentration value.   The values are shown in column 4 of Table 29.   The expected probit values Y are then converted to "working probit values" (y) by using the formula:

$$y = y_0 + kp,$$

where the values of y_0 and k are to be read from Fisher & Yates, Table XI,[1] corresponding to each Y and the adjusted mortality values are used as p.   (Values of y_0 and k corresponding to selected values of Y were shown in Table 25.)

The values of y at each concentration computed by this formula are given in column 5 of Table 29.

Table 29.   Basic data for computation of LD_{50}

Logarithm of concentration	Number of mosquitos	Adjusted percentage mortality	Expected probit (graphical)	Working probit	Auxiliary quantity	Weight
x	n	p	Y	y	x'	w
(1)	(2)	(3)	(4)	(5)	(6)	(7)
0.699	31	8.3	3.8	3.63	4.557	7.9
1.000	34	47.4	4.9	4.94	1.360	19.3
1.301	36	82.4	6.0	5.93	0.656	14.9
1.602	27	100.0	7.0	7.42	0.421	3.3

[1] Fisher & Yates use symbols of $Y - \frac{P}{Z}$ and $\frac{1}{Z}$ in place of our notation y_0 and k.

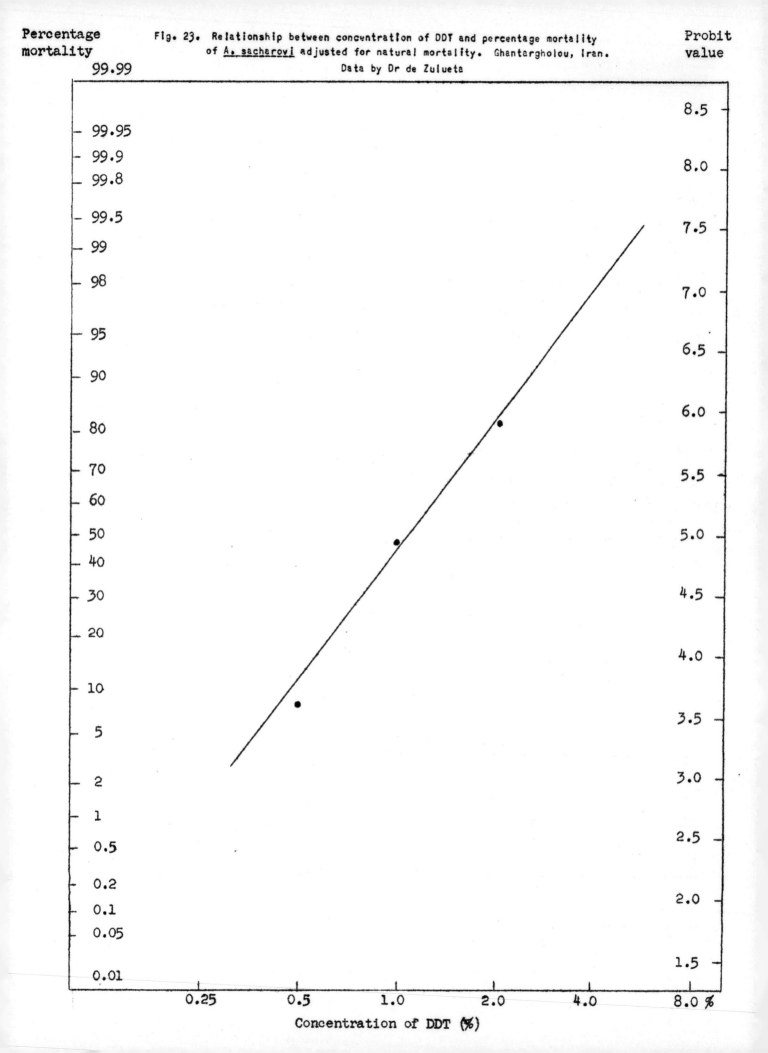

Fig. 23. Relationship between concentration of DDT and percentage mortality of <u>A. sacharovi</u> adjusted for natural mortality. Ghantargholou, Iran. Data by Dr de Zulueta

Percentage mortality

Probit value

Concentration of DDT (%)

The next step is to obtain an auxiliary value x' corresponding to each expected probit value Y; some of the values x' are shown in Table 30 below for the purpose of illustration. A detailed table is available in Fisher & Yates (1953) (Table XII). The values for our numerical example are shown in column 6 of Table 29.

Table 30. Values of auxiliary quantity x'

Y	x'
2.0	225.3
2.5	56.70
3.0	18.101
3.5	7.205
4.0	3.4770
4.5	1.9640
5.0	1.2533
5.5	0.8764
6.0	0.6557
6.5	0.5158
7.0	0.4214
7.5	0.3543
8.0	0.3046
3.8	4.5571
4.9	1.3599
6.0	0.6557
7.0	0.4214

Next we read the values of weighting coefficients from a ready-reckoning table (Fisher & Yates, Table XI, or Finney (1952) Table II). Selected values are shown in Table 31 below corresponding to the percentage natural mortality of 0%, 5%, 10% and 15%. The value of the weighting coefficient decreases as the natural mortality increases, for the reason that a portion of the mosquito mortality at different concentrations is to be regarded as due to natural causes and thus not all of the mosquitos used at each concentration contribute to the information on the toxicity of the insecticide. The weight to be assigned to each concentration is the weighting coefficient multiplied by the number of mosquitos tested at that level. Actual values of the weight (w) for various concentrations in our numberical example are shown in column 7 of Table 29.

Table 31.   Weighting coefficients when there is natural mortality

Expected probit Y	Natural mortality K			
	0%	5%	10%	15%
2.0	.01457	.00036	.00017	.00011
2.5	.04979	.00525	.00264	.00169
3.0	.13112	.03957	.02228	.01497
3.5	.26907	.15050	.10103	.07389
4.0	.43863	.32937	.25797	.20766
4.5	.58099	.49633	.42716	.36960
5.0	.63662	.57599	.52087	.47054
5.5	.58099	.53990	.50056	.46286
6.0	.43863	.41281	.38746	.36258
6.5	.26907	.25470	.24044	.22628
7.0	.13112	.12442	.11773	.11106
7.5	.04979	.04728	.04478	.04228
8.0	.01457	.01384	.01311	.01238
3.8		.25409		
4.9		.56921		

Next we compute the following quantities:

$$S_{xx} = Swx^2 - \frac{(Swx)^2}{Sw}$$

$$S_{xx'} = Swxx' - \frac{(Swx)(Swx')}{Sw}$$

$$S_{xy} = Swxy - \frac{(Swx)(Swy)}{Sw}$$

$$S_{x'x'} = Swx'^2 - \frac{(Swx')^2}{Sw} + \frac{n_c(100 - K_o)}{K_o}$$

$$S_{x'y} = Swx'y - \frac{(Swx')(Swy)}{Sw} + \frac{n_c(K_c - K_o)}{K_o}$$

where S denotes the summation of values.

In the next two formulae n_c denotes the number of mosquitos in the control group (i.e. 38 in our numerical example), and K_c is the observed percentage mortality of the control group. Another symbol K_o has been introduced, viz. the provisional value of the natural mortality. In our numerical example we have taken K_o to be 5.0% whereas the value of K_c was 5.263%.

Example:

Applying the above formulae to our numerical example, we first compute Swx, Swx', etc. (Table 32).

Table 32.   Computation of Snwx, Snwx', Snwy, etc.

x	x'	y	w	wx	wx'	wy	wx^2	wx'^2	wxx'	wxy	wx'y
0.699	4.557	3.63	7.9	5.52	36.00	28.68	3.86	164.05	25.16	20.05	130.68
1.000	1.360	4.94	19.3	19.30	26.25	95.34	19.30	35.70	26.25	95.34	129.67
1.301	0.656	5.93	14.9	19.38	9.77	88.36	25.22	6.41	12.72	114.95	57.96
1.602	0.421	7.42	3.3	5.29	1.39	24.49	8.47	0.58	2.23	39.23	10.31
Total			45.4	49.49	73.41	236.87	56.85	206.74	66.36	269.57	328.62

By using these values, the quantities are found to be:

$$S_{xx} = 56.85 - \frac{49.49^2}{45.4} = 2.90$$

$$S_{xx'} = 66.36 - \frac{49.49 \times 73.41}{45.4} = -13.66$$

$$S_{xy} = 269.57 - \frac{49.49 \times 236.87}{45.4} = 11.36$$

$$S_{x'x'} = 206.74 - \frac{73.41^2}{45.4} + \frac{38 \times 95}{5} = 810.04$$

$$S_{x'y} = 328.60 - \frac{73.41 \times 236.87}{45.4} + \frac{38 \times 0.263}{5} = -52.39$$

By using these quantities we then compute:

$$b = \frac{S_{xy} S_{x'x'} - S_{x'y} S_{xx'}}{S_{xx} S_{x'x'} - (S_{xx'})^2}$$

$$\frac{\delta}{100 - K_o} = \frac{S_{x'y} S_{xx} - S_{xy} S_{xx'}}{S_{xx} S_{x'x'} - (S_{xx'})^2}$$

$$a = \frac{Swy}{Sw} - b \frac{Swx}{Sw} - \frac{\delta}{100 - K_o} \frac{Swx'}{Sw}$$

Example:

$$b = \frac{11.36 \times 810.04 - (-52.39) \times (-13.66)}{2.90 \times 810.04 - 13.66^2} = 3.92$$

$$\frac{\delta}{100 - K_o} = \frac{(-52.39) \times 2.90 - 11.36 \times (-13.66)}{2.90 \times 810.04 - 13.66^2} = 0.00150$$

$$a = \frac{236.87}{45.4} - 3.92 \times \frac{49.49}{45.4} - 0.00150 \times \frac{73.41}{45.4} = 0.942$$

By applying the formula $Y' = a + bx$, we calculate new probit values (Y') corresponding to each value of x as shown below:

x	Y'	Y
0.699	3.68	3.8
1.000	4.86	4.9
1.301	6.04	6.0
1.602	7.22	7.0

The values of Y' are compared with those of empirical probit Y (column 4 of Table 29).   In our example it is seen that no appreciable differences exist between Y and Y'.   On the other hand from the quantity $\delta/(100 - K_o)$ computed above we find

$$\delta = 0.00150 \times (100 - 5.0) = 0.143 \ (\%)$$

The quantity δ is the amount of adjustment which we should add to our provisional estimate of the natural mortality. Thus our provisional value K_o being 5.0% our revised value should be 5.14%. However, since the above-obtained value of δ is very small no further adjustment is needed in the present case. Thus both the provisional value of the natural mortality and the provisional regression line are found to be close to the revised values. This being the case, the value of the logarithm LD_{50} is obtained by the formula:

$$Log\ LD_{50} = \frac{5 - a}{b}$$

In the present example,

$$Log\ LD_{50} = \frac{5 - 0.942}{3.92} = 1.035$$

Therefore LD_{50} = antilog 1.035 = 10.8.

In order to obtain the LD_{50} in terms of percentage concentration, we should divide this figure by 10, which provides us with the value of 1.08%.

In the present example the values of Y and Y' did not appreciably differ and the quantity δ was very small compared with the value of K_o. In cases where Y' is found to differ appreciably from Y or δ is not negligibly small, a second cycle of the procedure similar to above should be followed by treating the Y' values as if they were the values Y and the quantity $K_o + \delta$ as our provisional value of the natural mortality K_o.

2.21.6 Precision of LD_{50} and comparison of LD_{50} values

Since each estimate of the LD_{50} is computed from observations made on a limited number of mosquitos, the estimated value itself is associated with error which can be estimated from the same data. This estimate of error is then used to obtain the limits within which the true value of LD_{50} is expected to lie with 95% (or 99%) probability. Two limits, upper and lower, called the "confidence limits" are thus obtained. A simple procedure of completing the confidence limits for LD_{50} was discussed in connexion with a graphically estimated LD_{50} value (see section 2.21.4.3.)

This procedure is still applicable, as an approximation, to a numerically estimated value of LD_{50} if we treat the values of Y' as the ones graphically expected. For more rigorous formulae which can conveniently be applied to the case of a numerically estimated LD_{50}, reference should be made to Finney (1952). In a discussion of the estimated confidence limits within which the true value of LD_{50} lies, it is to be noted that the magnitude of the error is one that is expected to occur if the trial is repeated under similar conditions. But such variation in LD_{50} as may arise through different methods of handling mosquitos, through change in hibernation period or season at which the experiment is carried out, may indeed sometimes produce an enormous amount of variability for the same species of mosquitos in the same place. While, therefore, the statistical error calculated for any set of data is no doubt of value, it cannot be presumed that the two confidence limits obtained are the limits within which the value of LD_{50} will lie if a similar experiment were carried out at the same place at some other time or by some other individuals. Unless a series of LD_{50} values together with their confidence limits are examined for the same place at different periods of time, it may be hazardous to ascribe any statistically significant decrease in LD_{50} values to the development of resistance to the insecticide. The extent to which the insecticide may have brought about selection of the strain by the temporary elimination of the susceptible ones should also be kept in mind.

A statistical test of significance is available by which the difference between any two LD_{50} values may be tested. But, as stated already, the difficulty may lie not in regarding one value as significantly different from the other, but rather in ascribing this significant difference to any particular factor under study to the exclusion of some other unknown factors which may indeed have been operating at different times.

2.21.7 Design of the test

The object of each test should be to estimate LD_{50} with a desirable degree of precision, that is, to ensure that the range of the confidence limits within which the estimated LD_{50} lies is not greater than the one stipulated. It is of course possible by proper planning of the trial to ensure that the range of the confidence limits is as narrow as desired. In this connexion the factors which deserve special remark are:

1. The concentration levels, that is, how many concentrations should be taken at what levels.

2. The total number of mosquitos to be tested at each concentration level.

If from past experience we know approximately the whereabouts of the LD_{50} and other LDs, an experiment should be so designed as to cover a range around the guessed value of LD_{50}. The information provided by a test is the greatest when the concentration levels chosen are around the true LD_{50}, i.e. when they range from about LD_{15} to LD_{85}. The value of the information diminishes rapidly as the concentration of the insecticide falls outside these limits. Therefore, the concentration levels to be tested should preferably be chosen wide enough only to cover the range which would add to pertinent information.

The choice of the number of concentration levels also depends on how confident we are in our preliminary guess of the location of LD values. When we are fairly sure of its location, we may choose three or four concentration levels extending from say LD_{10} to LD_{90}. In the absence of such information a pilot test may first be carried out with only a few mosquitos at various trial concentration levels to get a rough idea of the LD values. The range should then be fixed wide enough so as not to miss the value of LD_{50} from that range. The concentration levels should be spaced at logarithmically equal intervals. For instance, if we are to cover a range of DDT concentration of 0.1 to 3.0% by using four concentration levels, the levels adopted may be 0.1, 0.3, 0.9 and 2.7%.

As far as possible, the total number of mosquitos may be divided equally for the test at each level. It is necessary to emphasize that the allocation or selection of mosquitos for test in different tubes should be made at random so that no bias from unknown sources of variation may vitiate the results. The larger the number of mosquitos at each level, especially around the LD_{50} value, the more precise the estimate would be. As far as practicable, the number of mosquitos tested at each concentration level should not be less than about 30.

2.22   Time Series, Trends, Seasonal and Cyclical Changes

Almost all malariometric indices, e.g. spleen rate, malaria morbidity or mortality rate, parasite rate, etc. are known to vary considerably not only according to seasons in a year but also from year to year.   When measurements are made at periodic intervals over the same population group for a number of years, the following types of variability can be studied.

1.   Variation associated with seasonal factors.

2.   Possible cyclical changes, i.e. a tendency for the rate or index to repeat itself at more or less regular intervals of a few years.

3.   Long-term trends or secular changes reflecting a gradual tendency towards a decrease or increase.

4.   Random variation arising from a multiplicity of unknown factors which superpose or interact with the factors described above.

If the effects of these possibly different causes of variation are of a strictly additive nature, i.e. if the effect of one factor on the index is not in any way interrelated with any of the others, simple statistical methods are sufficient to analyse and separate these effects.   Usually, however, there may be a considerable degree of interrelationship to the extent that the effect of one factor may not be confined to any single period, but may be carried forward and may in some cases altogether change the magnitude of the successive values.   All the same, it is of considerably interest to malariologists to study, maybe in a rough manner, what these various forms of variability are.   For this purpose the first step would be to plot these individual measurements by means of a line chart which would show at a glance the salient types of variation in the data.

2.22.1   Study of seasonal variation

From an examination of weekly, fortnightly or monthly figures, we can easily study the season or seasons during which malaria shows a tendency to increase. In the first place, it is preferable to tabulate figures for cases or deaths for a number of consecutive years, as in Table 33 below which gives monthly malaria deaths for Mysore State, India, for the period 1939-1947.

Table 33.   Mysore State, India.   Monthly deaths from malaria, 1939-1947

Year	Jan.	Feb.	Mar.	Apr.	May	June	July	Aug.	Sept.	Oct.	Nov.	Dec.	Total
1939	2966	2893	4342	3456	2563	2210	2268	2389	2279	2482	3241	3653	34 742
1940	3116	2466	2852	3144	2814	2909	2793	2517	2547	2646	2917	3411	34 137
1941	3249	2511	2819	2873	3011	2871	3151	2878	2955	3266	3460	3171	36 015
1942	3247	2591	2960	2783	2989	2212	2276	2414	2175	2626	2915	2786	31 974
1943	2532	2409	2628	2683	2323	2294	2628	2446	2475	2925	2909	3893	32 145
1944	3354	2836	2704	2832	3021	2924	3027	3229	3423	4074	4441	4691	40 556
1945	3840	2988	3561	2934	2987	2681	2636	2490	2432	2545	2690	2649	34 433
1946	2811	2265	1959	1839	1645	1640	1759	1591	1627	1841	1903	1910	22 790
1947	2132	1999	1802	1979	1957	2175	2067	2342	1962	2416	2686	2353	25 870
Median	3116	2511	2819	2832	2814	2294	2628	2446	2432	2626	2915	3171	
Adjusted median	3015	2690	2728	2832	2723	2294	2543	2367	2432	2541	2915	3069	

Since the number of days in different months varies it is desirable to adjust these monthly figures so as to bring them to a common base of 30 days.   Thus the figure for the month of February should be increased by multiplying by the fraction 30/28 (or 30/29), that for January reduced by multiplying by 30/31 and so on. These adjustments have been made to the median values.

The study of seasonal variation is facilitated by working out median values separately for each month and preparing a line chart of the median values shown in Fig. 24.   Two more curves showing the maximum and minimum figures (adjusted for variation in the number of days) are also drawn.   When the figures of the current month are plotted in a progressive manner on this chart it is easy to watch the extent to which an increase or a decrease over the normal is taking place. Such charts could be filled in month after month - or week by week if weekly data have been plotted instead of monthly data.   The charts may be drawn on semilog paper.

Malaria being essentially a seasonal disease, interesting studies on seasonal variation are provided by Iyengar (1932), and Wenyon (1921), who studied the seasonal variations in three species of malaria parasites, Barber & Mayne (1924) who studied the monthly malaria infections in infants to fix the transmission season, and Mayne (1928) who studied the seasonal variation of malaria infections in relation to relative humidity and the life-cycle of malaria parasite in the vector species.

2.22.2 Elimination of seasonal effect

One simple method of eliminating the effect of seasonal variability would be to study a figure calculated for the whole year. Although a calendar year is generally used for this purpose it is advisable to choose the year in such a manner that the period of seasonal rise and fall which may extend from one calendar year to another, is included. For instance, if it is known that the malaria incidence shows a tendency to increase in the month of July, reaching its peak by about December and declining to a low level again by the end of May, it would be advantageous to work out total annual index for the year beginning 1 June of one year and ending with 31 May of the next year. Such total annual figures, when plotted with respect to time, will then be free of seasonal variation and thereby enable us to study any tendency towards periodicity or a simple long-term trend.

2.22.3 Elimination of cyclical variability

Once the annual figures are charted with respect to time a rise and fall in the epidemics may be readily discernible to the eye. There may be a peak occurring at intervals of about six, seven or eight years approximately. If the series of observations extend over a long enough period, cyclical variation can be eliminated by means of what is called the "moving median" or "moving average". For this purpose, in the first instance, we first decide for how many years an average is to be worked out. If the mean period separating individual peaks occurs say approximately every seven years, we proceed by taking the median or average value of the figures for the first seven years and plotting a point on the same curve corresponding to the fourth year from the beginning. Next we leave out the value for the first year and calculate the median or average for the next seven years, that is second to the eighth year,

Fig. 24.   Mysore State, India.   Monthly median malaria deaths,
1939-1947

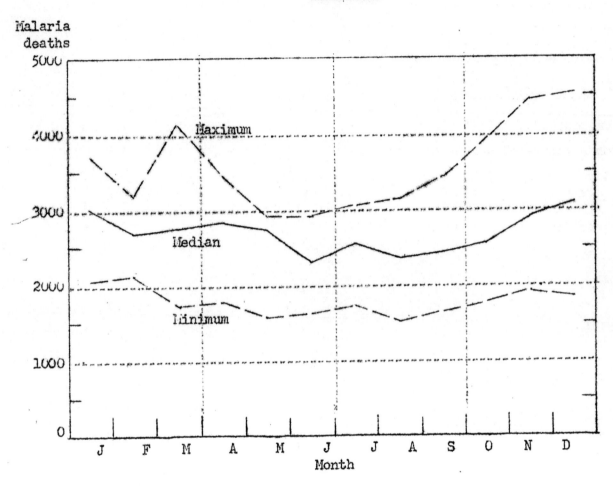

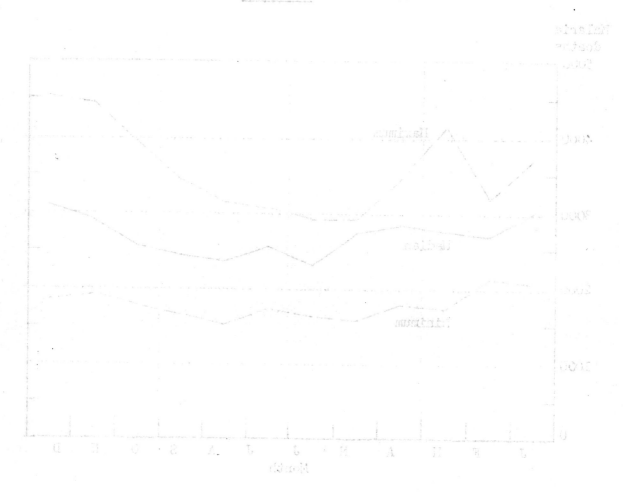

Fig. 24. Mysore State, India. Monthly median malaria deaths, 19..-19..

and plot this median or average at the fifth year.   Next we leave the first two
years and calculate the median or average for the next seven years (third to ninth),
and plot this median or average to correspond to the sixth year.   In this manner,
by successively leaving out one year in the beginning and including a new one each
time, we calculate the moving median or average values for each seven-year period
and obtain another line of plotted median or average values.   This curve of moving
medians or averages indicates in an approximate manner what the long-term trend is.

The following is an example of moving means applied to the data of epidemic
figures in the Punjab, India, from 1867 to 1943.   The original data (Yacob & Swaroop,
1945) and the three-year and seven-year moving averages are given in Table 34, and
are shown diagramatically in Fig. 25.   It is seen that by computing three-year
moving averages, the random fluctuations in the original data are considerably
reduced.   A possible cyclical variation with the period of about seven or eight
years is suggested.   By computing seven-year moving averages any such cyclical variation
is eliminated and the long-term declining trend is more clearly brought out.

We can work out the deviation of each year's value from the corresponding seven-
year moving median curve and plot the deviations (negative and positive) on a new chart.
These deviations will indicate the effect of cyclical variation on which of course
will be superposed the effect of other random factors.   The effect of random factors
may be reduced to some extent by working out a curve of moving means or medians by
taking only three successive observations each time.

Table 34.   Punjab, India.   Epidemic figures and moving averages, 1867-1943

Year	Epidemic figure	Three-year moving average	Seven-year moving average	Year	Epidemic figure	Three-year moving average	Seven-year moving average
1867	1.816			1906	2.008	1.529	1.995
1868	1.207	2.379		1907	1.505	2.767	1.901
1869	4.115	2.559		1908	4.788	2.605	1.841
1870	2.355	2.574	2.189	1909	1.521	2.508	1.855
1871	1.251	2.079	2.173	1910	1.215	1.170	1.784
1872	2.632	1.944	2.346	1911	0.774	1.054	1.758
1873	1.948	2.094	2.418	1912	1.173	1.154	1.231
1874	1.703	2.023	2.246	1913	1.514	1.336	1.266
1875	2.417	2.913	2.563	1914	1.320	1.312	1.443
1876	4.618	2.729	2.551	1915	1.103	1.395	1.400
1877	1.152	3.081	2.487	1916	1.761	1.774	1.448
1878	3.472	2.390	2.588	1917	2.457	1.563	1.349
1879	2.545	2.507	2.575	1918	0.470	1.478	1.343
1880	1.505	2.152	2.085	1919	1.508	0.935	1.383
1881	2.407	2.080	2.365	1920	0.826	1.204	1.407
1882	2.328	1.973	2.096	1921	1.278	1.161	1.268
1883	1.183	2.208	1.906	1922	1.380	1.530	1.401
1884	3.114	1.963	1.979	1923	1.932	1.599	1.447
1885	1.592	1.972	1.884	1924	1.485	1.606	1.472
1886	1.210	1.607	1.864	1925	1.400	1.572	1.431
1887	2.018	1.657	2.072	1926	1.830	1.409	1.489
1888	1.743	1.982	1.789	1927	0.997	1.274	1.389
1889	2.186	2.190	2.028	1928	0.994	1.259	1.367
1890	2.641	1.987	2.110	1929	1.787	1.338	1.382
1891	1.133	2.347	2.096	1930	1.233	1.449	1.373
1892	3.267	2.061	2.039	1931	1.326	1.239	1.398
1893	1.782	2.322	1.894	1932	1.159	1.532	1.409
1894	1.917	1.682	1.915	1933	2.112	1.481	1.297
1895	1.348	1.478	1.942	1934	1.173	1.452	1.260
1896	1.168	1.770	1.648	1935	1.071	1.084	1.184
1897	2.793	1.760	1.839	1936	1.007	1.017	1.158
1898	1.318	1.774	1.912	1937	0.974	0.925	1.036
1899	1.212	1.883	1.918	1938	0.794	0.915	1.051
1900	3.119	2.252	2.018	1939	0.978	1.008	1.260
1901	2.425	2.311	1.790	1940	1.253	1.170	1.327
1902	1.390	1.895	1.755	1941	1.278	1.689	
1903	1.870	1.485	1.869	1942	2.536	1.764	
1904	1.195	1.380	1.638	1943	1.477		
1905	1.075	1.426	1.976				

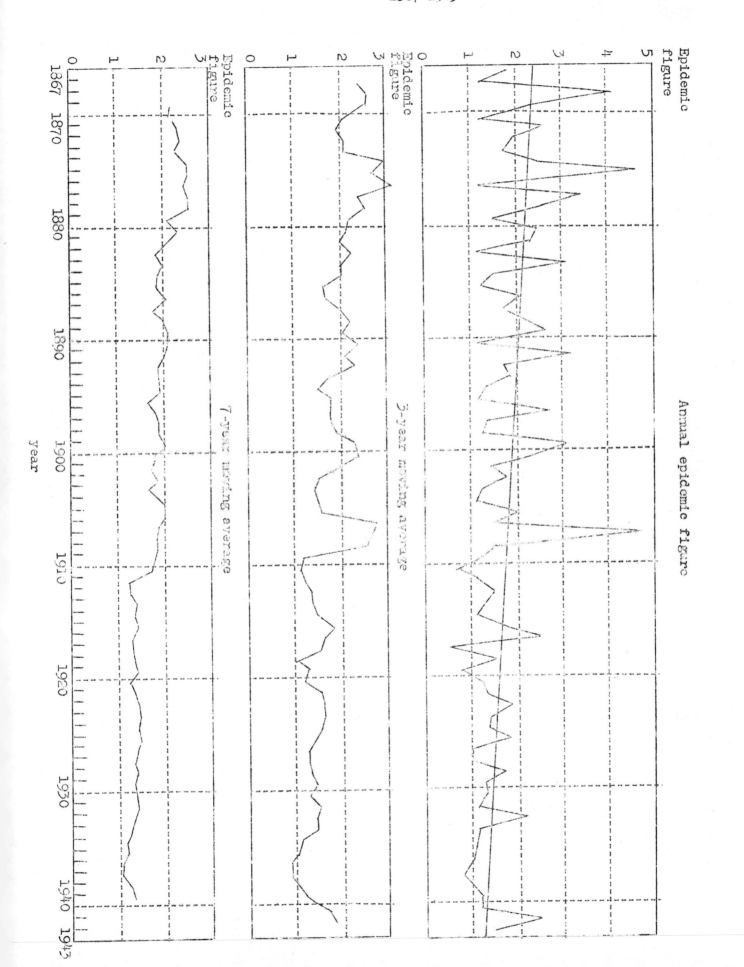

Fig. 25. Punjab, India. Epidemic figures and moving averages, 1367-1943

2.22.4   Fitting a trend line

When successive values of an index follow a trend which is more or less constant in its increase or decrease, a straight line to describe this trend may be fitted to the observed values.   The values of the annual epidemic figure recorded in the Punjab, India, discussed above (Table 34), would seem to show a decrease with time.   Fitting a straight line to these values would enable us to know the average annual rate of decrease.   The algebraic method used in fitting the line is called the method of least squares and the line thus fitted is called the "regression line".   Its equation is expressed as

$$y = a + bx$$

where x and y are the two variables, x denoting time and y the value of the index.

Thus, corresponding to each time x_1, x_2, ..., x_n, the observed values of the index would be y_1, y_2, ..., y_n, respectively.   In fitting a straight line we attempt to calculate the numerical value of the constants "a" and "b" so that the straight line best fits the observed data.

If $\bar{y}$ and $\bar{x}$ denote respectively the arithmetical means of the x and y series of values, then the desired values of a and b are given by the formula:

$$a = \bar{y} - b\bar{x}$$

$$b = \frac{\Sigma x_i y_i - n\,\bar{x}\,\bar{y}}{\Sigma x_i^2 - n\,\bar{x}^2}$$

where Σ sign indicates that the summation would extend over all the n values.

As an example we may work out the regression line which fits the annual epidemic figure data of the Punjab for the period 1867-1943, i.e. 77 years (n = 77).   For values of x we could have used the same figures as the years, but it facilitates the computation if as working values of x we take x_1 to be 0, for the year 1867, $x_2 = 1$ for the year 1868, $x_3 = 2$ for the year 1869, ..., and $x_n = x_{77} = 76$ for the year 1943.

The corresponding values of y are those shown in Table 34, and are:

$$y_1 = 1.816, \quad y_2 = 1.207, \quad y_3 = 4.115, \quad \ldots, \quad \text{and} \quad y_n = y_{77} = 1.477$$

The values of quantities in the formula are computed as follows:

$$\bar{x} = \frac{1}{n} \Sigma x_i = \frac{0 + 1 + 2 + 3 + \ldots + 76}{77} = \frac{2926}{77} = 38$$

$$\bar{y} = \frac{1}{n} \Sigma y_i = \frac{1.816 + 1.207 + 4.115 + \ldots + 1.477}{77} = \frac{135.567}{77} = 1.7606$$

$$\Sigma x_i^2 = 0^2 + 1^2 + 2^2 + 3^2 + \ldots + 76^2 = 149226$$

$$\Sigma x_i \, y_i = 0 \times 1.816 + 1 \times 1.207 + 2 \times 4.115 + 3 \times 2.355 + \ldots + 76 \times 1.477$$

$$= 4542.857$$

$$b = \frac{4542.857 - 77 \times 38 \times 1.7606}{149226 - 77 \times 38^2}$$

$$= -0.01600$$

$$a = \bar{y} - b\bar{x} = 1.7606 - (-0.01600) \times 38 = 2.3686$$

Therefore, the formula for the regression line is:

$$y = 2.369 - 0.016 \, x$$

The value of b is negative, thus indicating a decreasing trend with time in the value of y. Its magnitude shows the amount of decrease in the value of y due to a unit increase in the value of x. Thus, in our example we may say that the value of the epidemic figure showed a decrease of 0.016 per year according to the regression line.

Having worked out the equation of the line we can draw it by means of the co-ordinate of two points on this line. Thus:

$$\text{at } x = 0, \quad y = 2.369$$
$$x = 76, \quad y = 1.153$$

When these points are joined by a straight line, the trend estimated by the method of least squares is shown in the diagram as Fig. 25.

3.   VITAL AND HEALTH STATISTICS

The term "malariometry", i.e. the application of quantitative measures to the study of malaria, deals generally with such data and indices as relate to malaria morbidity, mortality, parasite rates, spleen rates and parasite density, etc., in so far as the human population is concerned, and in regard to the mosquito and parasite populations with several such indices as are mentioned in WHO Malaria Terminology (Covell et al, 1953).   Statistical information of this kind is normally collected by the malaria worker in the course of his work.   But there also exist other national and local sources of useful information which have more or less a direct bearing on the study of malaria.   Further, when the interest of the malaria worker is not confined to a relatively small or restricted community under his observation, but to the population at large, the facilities available to him for collecting statistical information for the entire population may be restricted. In this connexion it is necessary to remember that over large parts of the world national and local systems for the collection of statistical information bearing on births, deaths or disease as well as data bearing on economic and social conditions, have been established and that much of this information could well be made use of in discussions of the malaria problem.   The national or local agencies collecting this information are the public health departments, or the national statistical agencies working in close relationship with each other.   It would be well, therefore, for the malaria worker to get acquainted with other relevant statistics collected by or obtainable through public health departments which would be of use to him.   Some of the important sources of such information are briefly referred to in the following paragraphs.

3.1   Population

In most of the countries of the world, generally at intervals of 10 years, a count is made of the total number of individuals inhabiting each locality.   In addition to the actual count, information is also collected at the same time in respect of several characteristics of the population, such as age, sex, marital status, economic characteristics, e.g. nature of occupation, employment status,

educational characteristics, etc.   This is called the population census.   Population
censuses in different countries of the world have been carried out around the years
1930-31, 1940-41, 1950-51, etc.   Census figures showing the total population as
well as the populations by age and sex or by other characteristics, are published
for each country as a whole by United Nations in the Annual Demographic Yearbook,
issued each year by the Statistical Office of the United Nations, New York.   More
detailed information is published in national census reports.   But even the national
published information may not always be sufficiently detailed.   For instance, it may
not show the population of individual villages separately.   If such information is
required it could be obtained from the census office of the country concerned.   The
population census reports also discuss and describe the main population characteristics of different areas, which may have a bearing on a study of the malaria problem
or in connexion with the planning of malaria projects.

In many countries, following the population count, estimates are prepared from
year to year of how the population is changing.   In making such estimates account
is taken of the differences in the recorded numbers of births and deaths;   numbers
which constitute the accretion (or depletion) of the population following each census.

In connexion with malaria work, it is necessary to remember that during the
process of census taking all the houses in each locality are serially numbered if
they do not already bear a permanent number.

3.2   Vital Statistics

In order to serve demographic, legal and health purposes, most of the countries
of the world have established a nationwide system whereby each vital event that
occurs (birth, death, foetal death, marriage, etc.) in individual households has to
be reported to some government agent and recorded.   From these vital records
statistical information relating to the total number of births, deaths, foetal
deaths, etc., is regularly compiled and published at the international level in the
United Nations Demographic Yearbook and also in the WHO Annual and Monthly Epidemiological Vital Statistics Reports.   More detailed information is published by each
country in its national vital statistics reports issued annually and often at more

frequent intervals, such as monthly.   Of particular significance is the fact that while registering the event of death, the age, sex and the cause of death (as far as it can be ascertained) is also recorded.

In interpreting these figures it has to be borne in mind that their accuracy and completeness depend on the efficiency with which national and vital statistical services operate.   In many advanced countries of the world, highly accurate vital statistical information is obtained.   In the less developed countries there are errors from omissions and inaccurate statements.   Owing to the paucity of medical staff to diagnose the cause of death correctly, the information of cause of death is generally faulty.   Nevertheless, information on the total number of deaths is available and is of considerable value.   Inaccuracy is generally pronounced in the case of the record of age.   If these drawbacks are kept in mind, the information available from vital statistics sources can be of value in the study of trends in births, deaths, etc.

From these vital records, various indices to summarize the information and to study levels and trends are calculated and published by United Nations, WHO, and by the national statistical offices.   Some of the important ones of interest to malaria workers are briefly mentioned in the following paragraphs.

The two terms "vital statistics" and "health statistics" have come to acquire somewhat different connotations in recent years.   The term "vital statistics" relates to facts, systematically collected and compiled in numerical form, relating to or derived from records of vital events, viz., live births, deaths, foetal deaths, marriages, divorces, adoptions, legitimations, recognitions, annulments or legal separations (United Nations, 1953).

The term "health statistics" covers all statistical information required in connexion with the administration of health work.   Thus, while in its broad sense it would cover data on population, vital events, morbidity, health (including medical) work performed and health facilities available, in this document the term is taken to mean data needed by health workers, exclusive of population and vital statistics.

3.3   Indices Used in Vital and Health Statistics

3.3.1   Rates or ratios

In the interpretation of vital and health statistics use is made of the relationship of various frequencies or counts of such events to the size of the population in which these events occur.   Many types of relationship are used; the more common ones are described below.

No standard definition of the terms "rate" or "ratio" applicable in general to health work has been adopted.   The term "rate" has been defined in statistical literature in various ways.   The essential feature of a rate is that it is a relative number or a statement of numerical proportion prevailing between two sets of things, or is the quantity or degree of a thing measured per unit of another. For our present purpose, it is sufficient to state that vital or health statistics frequencies must be converted into relative numbers or rates by relating the absolute numbers to some base figure or "population".   What is necessary is that the population to which the events are related must correspond, or in other words, should be as nearly as possible, the actual population group in which the events occurred or the population exposed to the risk of the event recorded.

The numerator of the rate, that is, the number of vital events, should be defined according to (a) the character of the event in question, (b) the geographic area to which the event belongs, and (c) the time period within which it occurred. The population to which the events are related in computing a rate, i.e., the denominator, should "correspond" to the numerator in all these aspects.   The denominator is usually the population of the area which gave rise to the event, or some approximation to that population.   However, the population is usually not recorded continuously; in most countries it is recorded accurately only at the time of the population census, and may be estimated for the beginning and the middle of the calendar year.   The problem is to determine the population figure which best "corresponds" to the vital events.   Most annual rates are computed by using the population estimate referring to 1 July (mid-year population).   It sometimes happens that, as the result of a new census or some other fresh information, there is an abrupt change of considerable magnitude in the population estimates used for calculating vital rates. When presenting a table of vital rates over a series of years, during which such a discontinuity occurs, reference to the change should be made in a footnote. The table itself should show clearly the point of discontinuity, either by a thin ruled line or a definite space, separating the years before and after the change. Otherwise quite fallacious conclusions may be drawn about the rate of increase or decrease of vital rates.

Adherence to the principle of correspondence between the vital events and the population base requires that the two series of data - vital or health statistics and population census or estimate - be defined, classified and tabulated in exactly the same manner. For many reasons, it is not always possible to achieve this aim precisely, and as a result the numerator and the denominator are sometimes not exactly comparable. So long as the divergencies are recognized and acknowledged, the computed rates are useful for many purposes, but ignorance or disregard of lack of correspondence can result in meaningless or misleading rates. In malaria work in particular, where a wide variety of indices are used, the need for such caution is all the more to be emphasized as indeed has been done by Covell et al. (1953) on pages 29-41 of "Malaria Terminology".

Simply relating the number of vital events to the population would always result in a rate of less than unity. Therefore, for ease in understanding and recording, it is customary to multiply the proportion by a constant, which for most rates is 1000. Thus, vital rates are in general expressed as "per 1000 population". Exceptions to this are cause-of-death rates or specific morbidity rates, in which, because of the relatively small numerator (deaths from selected causes), and the large total population figure, the rates are usually calculated "per 100 000 of population".

3.3.2 Incidence or prevalence

There are three general types of information to be considered. The first concerns data on prevalence or the existence of a disease at a given point of time such as on a certain day. For instance, prevalence data would tell us what percentage of population was suffering from malaria at the time the survey was made. This type of data is usually collected by census methods and is called the "point prevalence data". The percentage of individuals suffering at any time, to the total population examined, is the "point prevalence rate".

The second general type of information called "incidence" refers to incidents or happenings which occur over a space of time, and of which a continuous record must be maintained in order to be complete. This includes occurrences such as births, deaths, and the appearance of new cases of disease in a defined period such as a year. New cases of malaria occurring during a year expressed as a rate per 1000 or 100 000 of the total population observed, would be an example of the incidence rate of malaria cases.

The third, of yet less general use, relates to the existence of disease among individuals during a period of time (period prevalence). This would include all those who were ill at the beginning of the period as well as new cases of illness during the period, irrespective of whether they recovered, died or continued to be ill till the end of the period. Period prevalence data are of considerable importance when dealing with such chronic diseases as cancer, tuberculosis, etc.

It is clear that to obtain information in these three categories different types of mechanism are required. By its nature, a survey is most effective in securing the point prevalence data, that is, we can go in and count the number of people, the proportion who are sick at the time, the number of houses and the proportion which were found sprayed, and data of a similar nature.

To obtain incidence data, one of the following methods must be employed:

(1) A system should exist in the community whereby each new occurrence is reported and recorded, as for instance the system for the registration of vital statistics.

(2) The collection, during surveys, of a history of occurrences previous to the survey. This is increasingly unreliable as events recede in time, and is most unreliable in primitive communities where survey data are most necessary.

(3)   The carrying out of repeated surveys in the same community, allowing
an estimate of change of situation during the interval, and therefore an estimate
of frequency of happenings.   A modification of this is a survey covering a considerable period of time, with repeated visits to given households and an opportunity to
observe what is happening in the interval.   This could be considered as a sort of
reporting system limited to a short time in a circumscribed area.

3.3.3   Definitions and formulae for calculating indices

3.3.3.1   Crude death rate

The crude death rate, which measures the decrease in a population due to death,
is perhaps the most widely used of any vital rate.   This is so for two reasons.
Firstly, it is relatively easy to compute, requiring only total deaths and total
population, and secondly, it has value as an index to numerous demographic and public
health problems.   It can be interpreted in terms of public health, since the rate of
death is the first approximate measure of the health status of a population.

The formula for the crude death rate is as follows:

$$\text{Annual crude death rate} = \frac{\text{Number of deaths which occurred among the population of a given geographic area during a given year}}{\text{Mid-year total population of the given geographic area during the same year}} \times 1000$$

As an example we may take the figures of two islands, Ceylon and Cyprus.
In 1950 there were 95 142 deaths in Ceylon and 3959 deaths in Cyprus.   From this
information, what can we say about the mortaility level of Ceylon in 1950 compared
with that of Cyprus?   Again, in Ceylon there were 91 889 deaths in 1949.   Does it
mean that in 1950 the mortality conditions of Ceylon were worse than in 1949?

The method of answering the above questions is by finding out what would have
been the number of deaths in the two places if they were both of the same population
size.   The population of Ceylon in 1950 was 7 544 000 and that of Cyprus in the
same year was 484 000.   In order to compare the mortality situation in the two

countries, we may ask the question: "How many deaths would have occurred in Ceylon and Cyprus if in both places the population was the same, as for instance 1000 persons?" The number of deaths per one thousand of the population of Ceylon can be calculated by the above formula:

Crude death rate per 1000 of the population of Ceylon =

$$\frac{95\ 142}{7\ 544\ 000} \times 1000 = 12.6 \text{ per } 1000$$

In the same way the number of deaths occurring in 1000 of the population of Cyprus $= \frac{3959}{484} = 8.2$ per 1000.

The above calculation shows that in Ceylon there were an average of 12.6 deaths in 1000 of its population, while in Cyprus there were only 8.2 deaths on an average in 1000 of the population.

We may adopt the same method to compare the mortality conditions of Ceylon in 1949 and 1950. There were 91 889 deaths in Ceylon in 1949, but the population of Ceylon in 1949 was less than that in 1950, being only 7 321 000. Therefore the number of deaths occurring in 1949 per 1000 of the population was: $\frac{91\ 889}{7\ 321} = 12.6$.

This calculation shows that the annual crude death rates of Ceylon in 1949 and 1950 were the same, so that the increase in numbers of deaths from 91 889 to 95 142 was in the same proportion as the increase in the population during the same period.

In the use of the crude death rate for inter-area comparisons, caution is necessary because mortality varies with age and, among other things, the crude rate which masks all differentials may be misleading, if the age-sex structures of the population being compared are not similar. Populations composed of a high proportion of persons at the older ages, where mortality is higher, will naturally show a higher crude death rate than a "younger" population.

Under most circumstances, the crude death rate is valid for comparisons for the same area from year to year, since changes in the composition of the population of an area occur rather slowly. If the time trend is studied for a long period of

years, the effect of population changes must be examined.   Greater caution is
necessary for comparisons between areas, since significant differences in crude
death rates may arise entirely from differences in the age-sex distributions of
the populations.   However, where it is known that the population distributions are
approximately similar, or where the crude rate differences are large, the crude rate
has great value as an index of mortality.

3.3.3.2   Age-specific death rate

Just as we calculate the crude death rate in a population, we can also
calculate the death rate for any specified section of the population.   A death
rate calculated in this way is known as a "specific" death rate, as distinct from
the "crude" death rate.   The formula for this useful type of death rate is as
follows:

$$\text{Annual death rate specific for age} = \frac{\text{Number of deaths which occurred among a specific age-group of the population of a given geographic area during a given year}}{\text{Mid-year population of the specific age-group in the given geographic area during the same year}} \times 1000$$

Example: The following Table 35 gives the mid-year estimated population in different
age-groups, the numbers of deaths occurring in the calendar year 1950 among the
undermentioned age-groups in Japan and the corresponding age-specific death rates.

Table 35.   Japan.   Population, deaths and death rates, by age, 1950

Age	Mid-year estimated population	Number of deaths	Age specific death rate per 1000
Under 5 years	11 150 000	223 946	20
5-9	9 560 000	19 998	2
10-14	8 710 000	10 339	1
15-19	8 530 000	21 472	3
20-24	7 710 000	36 124	5
25-29	6 160 000	33 096	5
30-34	5 190 000	26 600	5
35-39	5 060 000	28 364	6
40-44	4 490 000	29 503	7
45-49	4 000 000	34 082	9
50-54	3 390 000	40 465	12
55-59	2 740 000	48 533	18
60-64	2 290 000)		
65-69	1 760 000)	355 602	56
70-74	1 290 000)		
75 and over	1 040 000)		

The method of calculating each specific death rate separately is exemplified
below:

Specific death rates for the age-group under 5 years $= \dfrac{223\ 946}{11\ 150\ 000} \times 1000 = 20$ per 1000

Specific death rates for the age-group 5-9 years $= \dfrac{19\ 998}{9\ 560\ 000} \times 1000 = 2$ per 1000

The age-specific death rates when plotted on a graph would give us a U-shaped
curve (see Fig. 26).

These rates measure the risk of dying in each of the age-groups selected for
the computation.   Usually such rates are computed for the entire span of years,
and are further specified by sex, so that rates specific for age and sex are given.
The specificity by age and sex eliminates the differences which would be due to
variations in population composition in respect of these characteristics, and to
this extent, specific death rates from different areas can be compared.

Fig. 26.   Japan.   Age-specific death rate, 1950

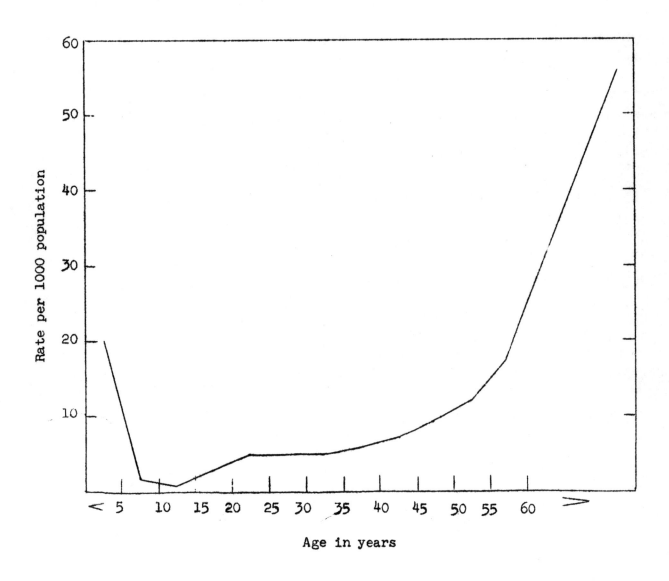

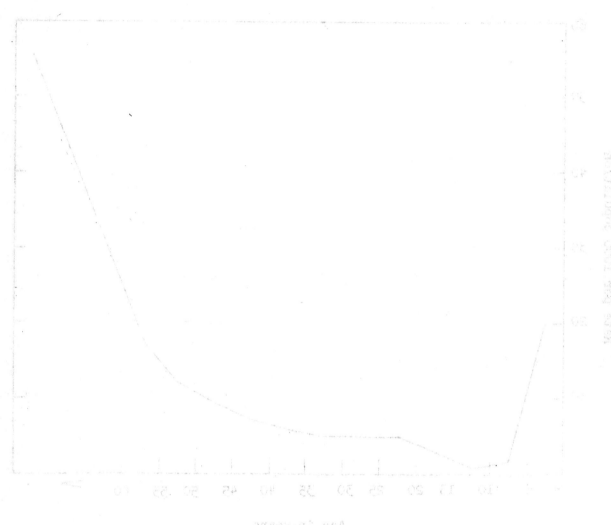

Fig. 26. Japan. Age-specific death rate, 1950

Age in years

Example: In Israel in 1944 there were 56 deaths among males and 60 deaths among females in the age-group 25-29 years.   The number of males in this age-group was 44 471 and the number of females was 38 427.   The specific death rate for males for this age-group 25-29 years

$$= \frac{56}{44\ 471} \times 1000 = 1.3 \text{ per } 1000$$

The specific rate for females in the same age-group

$$= \frac{60}{38\ 427} \times 1000 = 1.6 \text{ per } 1000$$

Age and sex are only two, although the most common, of the characteristics for which specific death rates are computed.   In each case, the essential requirement is that the events in the numerator must derive from a similarly defined population in the denominator, and that the two figures should refer to the same time period and to the same geographic area.

3.3.3.3   Infant mortality rate

The infant mortality rate is similar to the age-specific death rate for infants under one year of age, with the difference that in the calculation of this rate the number of live births occurring during the year in question is substituted for the population under one year of age.   The formula thus becomes:

$$\text{Annual infant mortality rate} = \frac{\begin{array}{l}\text{Number of deaths under one year of age which occurred among the population of a given geographic area during a given year}\end{array}}{\begin{array}{l}\text{Number of live births which occurred among the population of the given geographic area during the same year}\end{array}} \times 1000$$

Example: During 1950 the number of live births in England and Wales was 697 097. The number of deaths under one year of age during the same year was 20 817.   The infant mortality rate for England and Wales for 1950 therefore was

$$\frac{20\ 817}{697\ 097} \times 1000 = 29.9 \text{ per } 1000 \text{ live births}$$

Infant mortality rates can also be calculated separately for geographical subdivisions or for specific population groups, such as separately for each sex.

The use of the number of live births during the time period as the base for the infant mortality rate has the advantage that it immediately eliminates the dependence on the population census figure or population estimates to which other rates are subject. This means that the infant mortality rate can be computed for any group or for any time period, providing the number of infant deaths and live births are available for that area and time period. Infant mortality rates for small areas are possible, therefore, in spite of the lack of population estimates, and rates for parts of years can be computed without the use of adjustment factors.

The most serious errors in connexion with the infant mortality rate are probably those of definition and registration. Variations in the definition of a live birth and a stillbirth (late foetal death) may produce appreciable differences from one country to another. There is a tendency of varying degree to neglect to register as live births those infants who, though born alive, die immediately at birth, or very soon after. Thus, live births may be under-registered, while infant deaths are more completely registered - a situation which could result in infant mortality rates larger than the true ones. It has indeed been said that, even without saving any more infant lives, it is possible to lower the infant mortality rate merely by improving birth registration.

Since the infant mortality rate is of such value, especially in the field of public health, its correct computation and interpretation is important. In most countries, the great risk of death at ages under one year is not equalled again in the life span until very old age is reached. But in contrast to deaths at older ages, infant deaths are more responsive to improvement in the environment and in medical care. Hence, infant mortality rates serve as one of the best indices to the general "healthiness" of a society.

3.3.3.4 Neonatal mortality rate

Infant mortality can be studied in further detail by classifying infant deaths first by the age of the infant at death. In accordance with the WHO Regulations No. 1, deaths in the first year of life are to be classified by age as follows:

By single days for the first week of life,

    7-13 days,
    14-20 days,
    21-27 days,
    28 days up to but not including 2 months
    By single month of life from 2 months to 1 year (2,3,4...11 months)

Neonatal deaths are defined as deaths occurring under 28 days of age. A rate calculated by dividing neonatal deaths by the total number of live births in the corresponding place and period (multiplied by 1000) is called the neonatal death rate.

3.3.3.5   Late foetal death rate or stillbirth ratio

In view of the variety of definitions of the term "stillbirth" current in different parts of the world, WHO has recommended that the term "foetal death" be used rather than "stillbirth". WHO has adopted the following definition of the term "foetal death": "'Foetal death' is death prior to the complete expulsion or extraction from its mother of a product of conception, irrespective of the duration of pregnancy; the death is indicated by the fact that after such separation the foetus does not breathe or show any other evidence of life, such as beating of the heart, pulsation of the umbilical cord, or definite movement of voluntary muscles."

"Abortion" as applied to a product of conception has not been defined by WHO.

Foetal deaths occurring after the twenty-eighth completed week of gestation are described as "late foetal deaths".

"Stillbirth" is considered synonymous with late foetal death, that is, a death occurring after twenty-eight or more completed weeks of gestation.

The registration and reporting of foetal deaths is incomplete in widely varying degrees in different countries. The use of total registered foetal deaths in the numerator will therefore produce a rate which will be subject to greater variation between countries than a rate calculated on the basis of the more stable "late foetal death". This is the rate which would relate the number of late foetal deaths to the number of live births in the following formula:

$$
\text{Annual late foetal-death rate} = \frac{\begin{array}{l}\text{Number of foetal deaths of 28 or}\\\text{more completed weeks of gestation}\\\text{which occurred among the population}\\\text{of a given geographic area during a}\\\text{given year}\end{array}}{\begin{array}{l}\text{Number of live births which occurred}\\\text{among the population of the given}\\\text{geographic area during the same year}\end{array}} \times 1000
$$

Late foetal-death rates computed according to the above formula would also provide continuity with the commonly accepted "stillbirth ratios".

3.3.3.6 Cause-of-death rate

Another class of specific death rate that is of great importance is the specific death rate by causes of death. The term "cause-of-death" is defined as the morbid condition, or disease process, abnormality, injury or poisoning, leading directly or indirectly to death. The "underlying cause of death" rather than the direct or intermediate antecedent cause, is the one adopted as the main cause for tabulation of mortality statistics. The underlying cause of death is defined as:

(a)   the disease or injury which initiated the train of morbid events leading directly to death, or

(b)   the circumstances of the accident or violence which produced the fatal injury.

Rates computed for various underlying causes of death may be considered as a form of crude or specific rate according to whether thay are computed on the basis of the total population or a specific subgroup. Except for infant mortality by cause and some sex-specific rates, most death rates by cause are computed on total population. Thus the formula for the crude cause-of-death rate may be set forth as follows:

$$
\text{Annual cause-of-death rate} = \frac{\begin{array}{l}\text{Number of deaths from a specified}\\\text{cause which occurred among the}\\\text{population of a given geographic}\\\text{area during a given year}\end{array}}{\begin{array}{l}\text{Mid-year total population of the}\\\text{given geographic area during the}\\\text{same year}\end{array}} \times 100\ 000
$$

<u>Example</u>: There were 447 deaths from malaria in 1954 in Ceylon. The mid-year
estimated population of Ceylon for 1954 was 8 385 000. Therefore, the specific
death rate for malaria in Ceylon in 1954

$$= \frac{447 \times 100\ 000}{8\ 385\ 000} = 5.3 \text{ per } 100\ 000$$

We may calculate specific death rates by cause in each sex of the population
and also in each age-group of the population.

Since the numerators of the rates are often small frequencies, the above formula
uses a constant of 100 000 rather than the usual 1000.

In spite of the simplicity of its computation, the crude cause-of-death rate is
subject to a number of qualifications. Firstly, it disregards (as do all crude
rates) the age-sex composition of the population. Secondly, its principal component
is a characteristic - the reported cause of death - which is perhaps subject to the
greatest degree of reporting error, its reliability being governed by the type of
certification and the method of reporting, coding and classification of the underlying cause of death.

3.3.3.7   Crude live-birth rate

The simplest and most usual live-birth rate is the one which relates all the
live births which occurred among a given population to that population's total.
Such a rate is known as the "crude live-birth rate". The formula is as follows:

$$\text{Annual crude live-birth rate} = \frac{\text{Number of live births which occurred among the population of a given geographic area during a given year}}{\text{Mid-year total population of the given geographic area during the same year}} \times 1000$$

<u>Example</u>: There were 904 941 live births in Egypt in the year 1950. The mid-year
estimated population of Egypt for 1950 was 20 292 000. The crude birth rate per
1000 for Egypt for 1950

$$= \frac{904\ 941}{20\ 393\ 000} \times 1000 = 44.4 \text{ per } 1000$$

The crude live-birth rate is an index to the relative speed at which additions are being made to a population through childbirth, and as such is a composite measure of all the factors affecting natality in the population under study - the age composition, the economic level, and true fertility.

3.3.3.8 Rate specific for other characteristics

Death-rates specific for marital status, for occupation, for urban-rural residence, for ethnic or religious groups or for any other characteristic, may be computed by using a formula essentially the same as that set forth for the age-specific rate, substituting for "age-group" the "occupation", "religion", or "marital status" group as required. The essential element of the formula - and the one upon which the validity of the specific rate rests - is that the numerator and the denominator should correspond in terms of the characteristic, such as "occupation", for which the rate is specific. This means, as noted previously that the events in the numerator must derive from a similarly defined population in the denominator, and that the two figures must refer to the same time period and to the same geographic area.

3.3.3.9 Fatality ratio or case fatality rate

This rate is defined as the number of deaths from a disease recorded during a defined period divided by the number of new cases recorded during the same period.

3.3.3.10 Morbidity rate

The number of new cases of a specific disease occurring during a period can be expressed as a rate of the total population exposed to risk of the disease. For instance, annual malaria morbidity rate can be calculated from the annual cases of malaria by the following formula:

$$\text{Annual malaria morbidity rate} = \frac{\text{Total number of new cases of malaria}}{\text{Mid-year population exposed to risk}} \times 1000 \text{ or } 10\ 000$$

Example: In Ceylon the number of malaria cases during 1936 and 1954 were 2 947 555 and 29 655 respectively. The corresponding mid-year populations were 5 631 000 and 8 385 000.

$$\text{Annual malaria morbidity per 1000 for Ceylon, 1936} = \frac{2\ 947\ 555}{5\ 631\ 000} \times 1000 = 523$$

$$\text{Annual malaria morbidity per 1000 for Ceylon, 1954} = \frac{29\ 655}{6\ 585\ 000} \times 1000 = 4$$

Such annual malaria morbidity rates for Ceylon are shown for several years in succession in Table 2.

3.3.3.11 Expectation of life

On the basis of the recorded mortality experience of a population, an estimate is usually made of the number of years a newborn infant, or a person at any specific age, can expect on the average to live if mortality conditions remain the same through the remaining span of life. This is called the "expectation of life", and provides in summary form the effect of mortality on survival. It is denoted by the symbol e_x^o where the letter x denotes the age at which the expectation of life is estimated; thus for a newborn infant the expectation of life is denoted by the symbol e_o^o, for a child who has attained the age of 5 years expectation of life will be denoted by e_5^o. Expectation of life figures at specified ages separately by sex are given for various countries in the following table:

Table 36. Expectation of life at specified ages by sex
for various countries

Continent, country, period and sex		Expectation of life in years at age					
		0	1	5	15	30	60
AFRICA							
Belgian Congo	M	37.64	42.45	44.04	37.78	27.69	10.63
African population, 1950-52	F	40.00	44.14	45.87	39.58	29.78	12.27
Egypt, 1936-38	M	35.65	42.09	49.75	43.53	32.96	13.29
	F	41.48	48.14	58.33	50.11	38.23	16.26
Union of South Africa	M	50.70	54.29	53.05	44.29	32.72	11.97
Asian population, 1945-47	F	49.75	52.82	51.62	43.08	32.12	11.96
AMERICA, NORTH							
Mexico, 1940	M	37.92	44.43	48.55	41.34	31.00	13.35
	F	39.79	46.22	50.90	43.75	33.31	13.54
United States	M	66.6	67.6	64.0	54.4	40.5	15.9
White population, 1952	F	72.7	73.3	69.6	59.9	45.5	19.0

Table 36 (continued).

Continent, country, period and sex		Expectation of life in years at age					
		0	1	5	15	30	60
AMERICA, SOUTH							
Brazil	M	49.80	54.65	53.87	44.82	32.82	12.80
Federal District, 1949-51	F	55.96	60.35	59.98	50.88	39.01	16.60
Chile, 1952	M	49.84	56.83	55.64	46.90	34.79	13.99
	F	53.89	60.62	59.95	51.23	39.25	16.42
ASIA							
Ceylon, 1952	M	57.6	62.2	62.3	54.1	40.6	16.0
	F	55.5	58.9	59.7	51.6	39.3	14.9
China, Taiwan, 1935-40	M	41.08	47.61	49.48	41.23	29.68	11.28
	F	45.73	51.46	54.56	46.44	34.83	14.18
India, 1941-50	M	32.45	39.00	40.86	36.24	26.58	10.13
	F	31.66	37.30	40.91	36.56	26.18	11.33
Japan, 1953	M	61.9	64.3	61.8	52.6	39.3	15.0
	F	65.7	67.7	65.3	56.0	42.6	17.7
Korea, 1938	M	47.20	51.11	53.42	45.68	33.83	12.84
	F	50.59	54.47	56.71	48.95	37.65	14.83
Thailand, 1947-48	M	48.69	52.00	51.27	43.81	32.53	12.69
	F	51.90	55.20	54.30	46.80	35.44	14.20
EUROPE							
France, 1950-51	M	63.6	66.1	62.7	53.1	39.3	15.1
	F	69.3	71.2	67.8	58.2	44.1	18.1
Western Germany, 1949-51	M	64.6	67.8	64.5	55.0	41.3	16.2
	F	68.5	71.0	67.6	58.0	43.9	17.5
Netherlands, 1950-52	M	70.6	71.6	68.1	58.5	44.3	17.8
	F	72.9	73.5	70.0	60.2	45.7	18.6
Spain, 1940	M	47.1	52.4	52.6	44.0	32.8	12.4
	F	53.2	58.8	59.5	51.1	38.9	15.2
England and Wales, 1953	M	67.30	68.36	64.70	55.01	40.78	15.03
	F	72.44	73.19	69.51	59.75	45.28	18.49
Sweden, 1946-50	M	69.04	69.92	66.35	56.80	43.02	17.05
	F	71.58	72.08	68.42	58.73	44.57	18.03
OCEANIA							
Australia, 1946-48	M	66.07	67.25	63.77	54.28	40.40	15.36
	F	70.63	71.45	67.91	58.27	44.08	18.11
New Zealand, 1950-52	M	68.29	69.03	65.39	55.79	41.89	16.19
European population	F	72.43	72.90	69.23	59.47	45.06	18.53
Maori population	M	54.05	57.69	55.42	46.40	34.25	12.81
	F	55.88	59.08	56.61	47.59	35.11	14.41

3.4   Rates Calculated for Periods Other Than a Year

Vital or health statistics rates are generally calculated on an annual basis, one advantage is that a year is a unit of time having all the seasons included in it. Thus, crude death rate, birth rate, morbidity rate, etc., can be compared from one year to the next.   But if we calculate a death rate based on figures for the first three months of one year for one place and compare it with the similar rate calculated for, say, another three months of the same year for another place, the comparison will be vitiated because of different seasons of the year.

Nevertheless vital and health statistics rates are sometimes needed for periods other than one year.   For instance, when long-term trends are to be studied it is advantageous to calculate rates for five-year (quinquennial) or ten-year (decennial) periods.   On the other hand many rates are calculated on a weekly, monthly, quarterly or half-yearly basis to study variations in them during a year.

If a quinquennial rate is required, the total events that occurred in a five-yearly period should be divided by five to make the rate comparable with the annual rate:

$$\text{Quinquennial rate} = \frac{\text{Number of times the specified vital event has occurred during the entire period of five years}}{5 \times \text{population estimated at the middle of the five years}} \times 1000$$

Example: The following are the population estimates and the number of deaths for each year, for Japan, for the five years 1946 to 1950.   To calculate the annual crude death rate and the quinquennial death rate for Japan for 1946-50:

Year	Population estimated for mid-year	Number of deaths	Crude death rate per mille
1946	75 300 000	1 326 592	17.6
1947	78 000 000	1 138 238	14.6
1948	80 200 000	950 610	11.9
1949	82 200 000	945 444	11.5
1950	82 900 000	904 876	10.9
Total		5 265 760	

$$\text{Quinquennial death rate of Japan} \atop \text{for period 1946-50} = \frac{5\ 265\ 760}{80\ 200\ 000} \times \frac{1000}{5} = 13.1 \text{ per mille}$$

We can calculate the decennial rate also in the same way as the quinquennial rate, the total deaths in this case being divided by 10 to arrive at an average annual figure.

$$\text{Decennial rate} = \frac{\text{Number of deaths in 10 years}}{\substack{\text{Estimated population at the}\\ \text{middle of the 10-year period}}} \times \frac{1000}{10}$$

It is to be noted that the denominator of the quinquennial death rate is the estimated population at the middle of the third year and that of the decennial death rate is estimated population at the end of the fifth year.

The rates calculated for periods shorter than a calendar year, such as for weeks or months, are also made comparable to the annual rate. The weekly rate, for example, is calculated by first multiplying the number of occurrences of one week by 52, in order to reduce it to an annual basis. This figure is then divided by the mid-year estimated population and the ratio is then multiplied by 1000.

$$\text{Weekly rates} = \frac{\substack{\text{Number of vital events occurring}\\ \text{in 1 week} \times 52 \times 1000}}{\text{Total mid-year estimated population}}$$

Similarly, monthly rates are calculated by first multiplying the number of events occurring in one month by 12 and then dividing by the mid-year estimated population and finally multiplying by 1000.

$$\text{Rate for January} = \frac{\substack{\text{Number of times the event has}\\ \text{occurred in January}}}{\text{Mid-year estimated population}} \times 12 \times 1000$$

Since the number of days in different months vary, it is preferable to multiply by the figure 365 and divide by the number of days in the month, i.e., 31 for January, 28 (or 29 for Leap year) for February, etc.

Quarterly or half-yearly rates are similarly calculated by reducing the figures to an annual basis and always using the mid-year estimated population as the denominator.

$$\text{Quarterly rate} = \frac{\substack{\text{Number of events occurring in a}\\ \text{quarter of the year} \times 4 \times 1000}}{\text{Mid-year estimated population}}$$

$$\text{Half-yearly rate} \quad = \quad \frac{\text{Number of events occurring during half-year period x 2 x 1000}}{\text{Mid-year estimated population}}$$

3.5 Certain Vital Statistics Rates for Selected Countries

In order to enable malaria workers to compare the vital statistics rates recorded for their areas with those normally observed, a few figures actually reported in recent years are given in the two tables below. The figures have been taken from the WHO Annual Epidemiological and Vital Statistics, 1954. Table 37 gives figures for large-sized countries. Even though they are of considerable interest, these figures do not bring out the possible range of variation existing among figures of small localities of the size for which malaria workers may assemble their data. For this reason Table 38 gives similar data for some territories of relatively small size.

Table 37.   Vital statistics rates for certain countries, 1954.

Country	Mid-year estimated population	Crude birth rate per 1000 population	Crude death rate per 1000 population	Infant mortality rate per 1000 live births	Neonatal mortality rate per 1000 live births
AFRICA					
Algeria (Moslem population)	8 405 000	43.2	13.7	85.7	**
Egypt (Localities with Health Bureau)*	9 396 000	48.5	22.4	178.6	35.3
AMERICA					
Canada	15 168 000	28.7	8.2	31.8	19.3
Chile	6 597 000	33.6	12.8	124.7	41.7
Mexico	28 850 000	46.4	13.1	80.5	29.1
United States	161 183 000	24.9	9.2	26.6	19.1
ASIA					
Ceylon	8 385 000	36.2	10.4	72.0	43.1
Federation of Malays	5 889 000	43.8	12.2	83.1	30.2
Japan	88 200 000	20.1	8.2	44.6	24.1
Union of India (Registration area)	233 033 000	25.8	13.1	114.2	**
EUROPE					
Denmark	4 406 000	17.3	9.1	26.9	18.0
England and Wales	44 274 000	15.2	11.3	25.5	17.7
France	42 951 000	18.9	12.1	40.7	21.6
Italy	47 800 000	18.3	9.2	53.0	27.3
Netherlands	10 615 000	21.6	7.5	21.1	14.7
Portugal	8 693 000	22.7	10.9	85.5	29.7
Spain	28 751 000	20.0	9.1	54.2	**
Sweden	7 214 000	14.6	9.6	18.7	13.8
Switzerland	4 927 000	17.0	10.0	27.2	19.9
OCEANIA					
Australia	8 989 000	22.5	9.1	22.5	16.2
New Zealand	2 095 000	25.8	9.0	24.1	14.9

* 1953

** Not available

From: WHO Annual Epidemiological and Vital Statistics, 1954

Table 38. Vital statistics rates for certain small-sized territories, 1954

Territory	Mid-year estimated population	Crude birth rate per 1000 population	Crude death rate per 1000 population	Infant mortality rate per 1000 live births	Neonatal mortality rate per 1000 live births
AFRICA					
Seychelles	37 000	32.3	12.2	58.7	24.0
Mauritius	530 000	41.3	16.0	81.1	**
AMERICA					
Bahamas	90 000	38.2	10.5	38.6	**
Barbados	225 000	33.7	11.3	109.4	36.2
British Honduras	77 000	42.0	11.4	93.5	40.9
Panama, Canal Zone	39 000	44.2	6.8	27.9	**
Virgin Islands (US)	24 000	36.6	12.5	38.7	22.8
ASIA					
Aden (Colony only)	140 000	24.4	11.6	156.6	38.3
Cyprus	514 000	27.0	7.2	52.0	27.4
Sarawak	602 000	25.1	7.7	75.6	27.4
EUROPE					
Isle of Man	56 000	11.2	14.8	16.0	11.2
Liechtenstein	14 000	22.4	8.8	43.3	**
Luxembourg	306 000	16.3	11.4	43.8	23.6
Malta and Gozo	320 000	28.1	9.6	67.0	33.1
OCEANIA					
American Samoa	21 000	36.4	5.9	29.7	9.0
Fiji	328 000	40.2	9.5	48.8	19.5
Guam	35 000	58.0	8.2	40.9	26.8
Hawaii	522 000	31.0	5.7	22.4	17.0
Tonga	52 000	40.1	6.0	58.7	**

** Not available

From: WHO Annual Epidemiological and Vital Statistics, 1954

3.6 Standardization of rates

The crude death or birth rates of two places cannot be regarded as strictly valid bases for comparison when the population of the two places have different age compositions. This point is illustrated by a hypothetical example of comparing three areas, A, B and C, for which the specific death rates by age are given in Table 39, together with the corresponding populations.

Table 39. Hypothetical data to illustrate need for standardization of rates

Age-group	Death rates per 1000			Population in thousand			Deaths at each age		
	A	B	C	A	B	C	A	B	C
(1)	(2)	(3)	(4)	(5)	(6)	(7)	(8)	(9)	(10)
0 - 14	15	16	17	4 000	3 500	3 000	60	56	51
15 - 29	10	11	12	2 000	3 000	3 500	20	33	42
30 - 44	14	15	16	1 500	2 000	2 500	21	30	40
45 & over	40	45	50	2 500	1 500	1 000	100	68	50
All ages	20.1	18.7	18.3	10 000	10 000	10 000	20.1*	18.7*	18.3*

* Crude death rate per 1000 population

It is clear from columns (2) to (4) that at each age-group area A enjoyed the lowest death rate; area C experiencing the highest. The crude death rates shown at the bottom of the columns (2) to (4) on the other hand, lead to contradictory conclusions inasmuch as the crude death rate of area A is shown as the highest. This fallacious conclusion arises owing to marked differences in the age composition, area A having the largest proportion of old people. It is clear, therefore, that an area which has a proportionately larger number of adult persons would have a lower crude death rate than an area with a large proportion of people in the very old and very young age-groups, even though the specific death rates in individual age-groups are higher in the former area. In order to compare the overall death rate of these two places, we should ascertain how much the difference in the two rates is due merely to the unfavourable age distribution of one area in comparison with that of the other. One method that has usually been adopted for this purpose is to calculate what would have been the death rates of the two populations if the age compositions of both areas were the same. This method is known as the direct method of standardization and can be illustrated by a worked out example, relating to the mortality experience in Ceylon and Ireland in the year 1951.

The crude death rates of Ceylon and Ireland were 12.9 and 14.3 respectively. This may lead us to believe that mortality conditions were more unfavourable in Ireland. As is shown below, this is not so. The age specific death rates as well as populations by age are shown for both countries in Table 40.

Table 40.   Specific death rates and population by age-groups for
Ireland and Ceylon, 1951

Age-group	Specific death rate per 1000 population		Population by age-group 1951		Standard population
	Ceylon	Ireland	Ceylon**	Ireland***	
Under 1 year	81.9*	46.0*	187 000	63 557	23 000
1 - 4 years	25.7	2.6	815 000	249 275	95 000
5 - 9 "	4.8	0.8	943 000	281 043	108 000
10 - 14 "	1.6	0.7	937 000	260 935	105 000
15 - 19 "	2.1	1.3	792 000	241 182	92 000
20 - 24 "	3.6	2.0	746 000	202 172	82 000
25 - 29 "	4.2	2.5	671 000	198 421	77 000
30 - 34 "	4.7	2.7	523 000	191 566	66 000
35 - 39 "	5.4	3.7	545 000	200 916	69 000
40 - 44 "	6.0	4.5	375 000	180 326	55 000
45 - 49 "	7.8	6.4	371 000	160 915	51 000
50 - 54 "	11.4	10.7	228 000	162 986	42 000
55 - 59 "	13.5	15.7	190 000	128 848	34 000
60 - 64 "	21.3	25.1	152 000	122 060	30 000
65 - 69 "	35.0	39.6	108 000	107 548	25 000
70 - 74 "	58.6	65.7	72 000	100 116	22 000
75 - 79 "	80.4	111.4	42 000	64 555	14 000
80 - 84	145.1	183.2	26 000	30 887	7 000
85 and over	325.1	272.6	19 000	13 285	3 000
All ages	12.9	14.3	7 742 000	2 960 593	1 000 000

*   per 1000 live births

**   mid-year estimate

***   census of 8 April

If, for the sake of argument we presume that the population of Ceylon was distributed
by age like that of Ireland, we can calculate the total number of deaths and the crude
death rate expected in Ceylon on this presumption. For this purpose we apply the
Ceylon death rate to the Ireland population in each age-group and calculate the
expected number of deaths. For instance, in the age-group 1-4 years, the population
of Ireland was 249 275 which, on the basis of the Ceylon specific death rate of 25.7
gives the total number of deaths as $\frac{249\ 275 \times 25.7}{1000} = 6406$ deaths. In the same manner
expected deaths are worked out for each of the other age-groups, the total expected
deaths being 49 585 which, divided by the population of Ireland, gives a death rate
of 16.7. We can now argue that if by age the Ceylon population was distributed as
in Ireland, the death rate in Ceylon would have been 16.7 compared with 14.3 in
Ireland.

We could just as well have applied the Irish mortality experience (age specific
death rates) to the Ceylon population by age-groups. In that case it is found that
in Ceylon the Irish specific mortality rates yield a death rate of 7.3 as compared
with a crude death rate of 12.9 recorded for Ceylon. The Irish death rate would be
lower than the crude death rate for Ceylon if the population distribution by age were
the same as in Ceylon. These two figures are comparable because the age distribution
has been taken to be the same for both countries.

It is customary when comparing two areas to standardize the rates by applying
the age specific death rates to a common population. For comparative purposes we
need not have applied the Ceylon specific death rates on the Irish population or
vice versa but taken yet another age distribution, as for instance an average of both
the Irish and Ceylonese figures, as is shown in the last column of the above Table.
This may be regarded as a standard population for purposes of comparison. The age
specific death rates for both Ceylon and Ireland would then be applied separately to
the standard population and a crude death rate worked out as has been done below.
The death rates for Ceylon and Ireland standardized on a common age structure are
found to be 14.1 and 10.8 respectively. The conclusion to be drawn from these two
rates is obviously different from that we would be lead to if only the two crude death
rates were compared. These standardized death rates for Ceylon and Ireland are
comparable because the population age distribution is the same.

Such standardized death rates are not normally published because of a lack of agreement on the choice of standard populations, but the principle of standardization is important and could be applied when comparing figures of two or more localities with varying age or sex composition.   The principle can of course be applied to any other specific rates, as for instance the malaria mortality or morbidity rates.

4. MALARIOMETRY

4.1 General Consideration

Malaria projects may be classified broadly into two groups:

(a) Malaria control or eradication demonstrations intended to establish the efficacy of modern methods in certain areas of high malarial endemicity, at the lowest feasible cost. These, in fact, are projects of current practice intended as public health measures to fight malaria by proven methods.

(b) Experimental or research projects to ascertain the efficacy of two or more antimalarial techniques or treatments. These are generally pilot projects intended to study and assess factors or results of some specific measures.

In order therefore that the final results should be scientifically sound and acceptable by public health administrators, the project should provide for careful collection of numerical facts. It is further implied that the statistical data so collected must be analysed by means of proper techniques and that the statistical significance of the results should be tested so as to disentangle, or make proper allowance for variation brought about by uncontrolled or uncontrollable factors. An important consideration to be kept in mind is that the project should be planned on a sufficiently large scale for the efficacy of the malaria control measures to be assessed with the necessary precision and for important differences if any between treatments to emerge into statistical significance.

Statistical methods are tools for the proper analysis and evaluation of results. Their aim is to ensure that different workers trying to interpret the same mass of figures arrive at similar or uniform conclusions. No statistical method can introduce any refinement or accuracy into the original data if in the first instance they are erroneously collected, or if they suffer from initial bias arising from faulty planning of the experiment. On the other hand, if a series of related measurements are available on the effect of different factors, statistical techniques may help in revealing the relationships where they exist. For these reasons it is of the utmost importance that careful thought should be given as to what numerical information should be recorded, how different sources of bias may be kept in check, and what are the different factors which are likely to produce variation in the final results, so that numerical data are collected to assess their relative importance.

From the statistical point of view, one has to think of the malaria problem as the resultant interaction of three well-known and distinct types of population:

(a) The population of human beings sub-divided into such categories as infected and uninfected, treated or untreated or classified by age, sex, occupation, economic status, housing and environmental conditions and the availability of medical relief, antimalaria or general public health measures.

(b) The population of anopheline mosquitos, of which the species may vary from place to place, according to season or year, and may be further affected by control measures directed against its larval or adult stages.

(c) The population of malaria parasites, whose multiplication takes place in both mosquito and man, and which can be sub-divided into the well-known four different species.

While man and mosquito can exist independently of each other, the parasite can exist and multiply only in either man or mosquito. Their population is therefore dependent on the numbers of mosquitos and men. In each locality these three populations may be variable from time to time, and the last two vary much more so than the first. The variation in human population would arise from births, deaths and migration, dependent upon facilities of communication, season, employment of labour, economic and social conditions. The variation in all three may be related to topography, availability of water, soil fertility, presence of other diseases, climatic conditions and communicability of disease in general and possibly other factors.

First attempts to resolve mathematically these complex interrelationships were made by Ronald Ross (1916). His work has been considerably advanced in recent years by Macdonald who, in a series of papers, has attempted to interpret by means of mathematical analysis the processes involved in the transmission of malaria. An elaboration of Macdonald's work is beyond the scope of this document. Special reference may, however, be made here to his paper on a new approach to the epidemiology of malaria, written in non-mathematical language "attempting to expose the methods of work used and show how the products of mathematical analysis can be used to elaborate understanding of the normal epidemiology of malaria in the field" (Macdonald, 1955).

The factors which can bring about variability in malaria incidence, therefore, are the human factor, the mosquito factor, the parasite factor, the environmental and social factors, topography, climate, communicability and preventive action. There is no doubt that the final picture of malaria incidence in any locality can be a highly variable one from season to season and from year to year over a number of years except in holoendemic situations.

These points must be constantly kept in mind when the effect of any specific measure such as DDT spraying is to be judged on the basis of recorded data. When arriving at such a judgement the statistician's first concern is to ascertain what the degree of variability in malariometric indices would have been before and after the application of DDT, if hypothetically no DDT was offered to the population of that area.

For instance, if owing to lack of clear understanding of the seasonal variation expected in that particular year, DDT happened to be offered at the time of the peak of malaria season, a subsequent reduction in mosquito population or malaria cases or parasite rates could not be ascribed solely to DDT, for the simple reason that a decrease in the incidence of malaria would have occurred in any case from natural causes. For the same reason, if antimalaria operations were carried out during an epidemic year, a reduced incidence in the one, two or more post-epidemic years could not legitimately be ascribed entirely to any specific measures.

A knowledge of the changes occurring in the three different populations from month to month and from one year to another may therefore be an important pre-requisite for any subsequent evaluation. The results of antimalaria activities cannot and should not, therefore, be evaluated merely by obtaining through a single preliminary survey of the area certain malariometric indices against which to compare indices in the post-operational period. While a preliminary survey is necessary for several other reasons, its value for statistical evaluation of results is limited, because it indicates levels at only one instant of time and fails to give indications of the expected direction (towards increase or decrease) in malaria incidence. In later sections, these points are further emphasized and the suggestion is made that inferences should be drawn by relying more on clear changes recorded in post-operational years relatively to the trend which existed before the campaign was initiated, than by single comparisons with data relating to one or two years prior to the campaign.

Sometimes, as an alternative, a check area (untreated) is selected near the experimental area to study simultaneously changes taking place in both the areas. The establishment of a check area for purposes of evaluation may not prove altogether satisfactory unless we possess additional data to show that, in both areas, malariometric indices would have varied from season to season and from year to year in a similar fashion, and if we are further assured that there is no time lag in the variation of indices of the two places, i.e. the changes in one area do not arise after a certain specific period, in comparison with the other area. A check area close to the experimental area may be affected by the control measures while if situated at some distance may indeed be quite different for unknown reasons. The one question which therefore generally remains unsettled from the statistical point of view is: is the check area a good control on the experimental zone? Or, have natural conditions been so dissimilar in the two areas as to produce different types of incidence or variability in them? In the latter case periods favourable or unfavourable for the spread of malaria in one zone will not correspond to similar periods in the other. This point could be verified by first finding long-term trend lines relating to malariometric indices of both areas, and separately working out fluctuations of the actual indices around the respective trend lines. If the corresponding fluctuations of the two areas show high degrees of positive correlation, (see section 2.19), the indication could be that natural conditions in the two zones were similar, and that any significant difference in the long-term trends after malaria operations was possibly due to malaria control measures.

An illustration of this idea is given in the work of Howard et al. (1935) who analysed monthly trap catches in Luquillo (Puerto Rico) from July 1927 through June 1932.

The areas were divided into inside and outside zones. Experimental measures were employed only in the inside zones. Thus, outside zones situated as near as possible to the inside zones but beyond the limits of the work, served as the check. It was admitted that the activities in inside zones probably had some effect on the "outside" due to overlapping of mosquito flight ranges; a factor which could not be allowed for. It was argued that although such an effect which might be expected to follow mosquito control work may be inconsiderable in comparison with the difference between the two zones, the blurring of differences would tend only to obscure and not exaggerate any beneficial effects of the work.

The seasonal variation of mosquito trap catches was first determined by estimating trends of the averages of the five points for each calendar month. The deviations were then calculated from this trend for each month, which expressed the effect of breeding condition without regard to the season. To these fluctuations, which are shown separately for inside and outside zones, trend lines were fitted as shown in the chart below (Fig. 27). In order to study whether the outside zone served as a good check on the inside, the deviations around the respective trend lines were correlated. The coefficient of correlation was found to be +0.521, which though not very high, is statistically significant, indicating thereby that a fair degree of correspondence existed between the inside and outside zones. The difference in the slopes between the two trend lines for the inside and outside zones was found to be statistically different, thus indicating a significant decline in the inside zone.

Owing to the interaction of several factors, malariometric indices would fluctuate considerably in the pre- and post-operational periods, and for statistical purposes it is of the utmost importance to ascertain what the amount of this expected fluctuation is in different areas, and whether or not these fluctuations occur in sympathy or independently in the experimental and check areas. When past experience is lacking, as is generally the case in under-developed areas, it may

Fig. 27 <u>Long-term trend of mosquito trap catches after elimination of seasonal variation for the inside and outside zones of Luquillo (Puerto Rico), 1927-1932*</u>

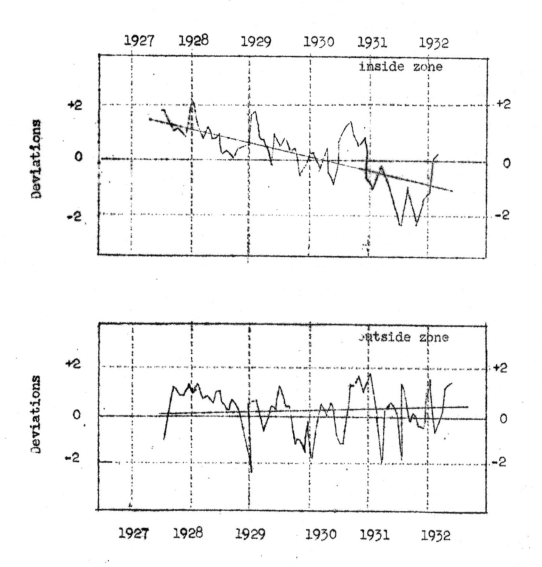

* Howard, Earle, and Muench, (1935)

seem virtually impossible to claim that the check areas were similar or would have
behaved similarly to the experimental areas.   This difficulty can be overcome if
we choose a group of say ten similar population units of reasonable size not
necessarily as large as the total experimental area and then select at random
(i.e. by casting lots) five of these population units for purposes of treatment
leaving the other five to serve as the check.   The desirable size of each such unit
will depend upon what malariometric units or indices are to be used in the final
evaluation.   This point is discussed in the next section.   If this scheme is
adopted then the five experimental villages and the five check villages will
separately give malariometric indices varying among themselves.   The within-
variation of each of these five values of any specific index will then provide us
with an idea of how much variability in that index was to be expected from
uncontrollable factors alone.   In other words we then possess a yardstick for
assessing the significance of the subsequent difference observed between the
average values of the index for the experimental and check areas.   This suggestion
therefore amounts to providing data in respect of the check area within the
experimental area, thus doing away altogether with the establishment of a separate
check area.

The above scheme is of course one that satisfies statistical considerations
and in actual practice could be considered suitable in such cases as the carrying
out of field chemotherapeutic trials.   It is however recognized that when
experimenting with residual insecticides where the result is judged by the
interruption of malaria transmission, this scheme of using individual villages as
units may not in many cases be suitable from the practical point of view.   This
is because of the possibility of people from the sprayed villages going for the
night into the neighbouring comparison villages or infected mosquitos possibly
emigrating from the comparison villages into the experimental ones.   Both these
factors will tend to mask the beneficial effect of residual spraying as judged
from the point of view of interruption of malaria transmission.   In this case we
are, as it were, interested in keeping the experimental village in isolation to
study the success of interrupting malaria transmission.   It is also necessary to

draw distinction between a project planned purely for the purpose of malaria
eradication from an area or one designed specifically to test strictly on
statistical considerations the comparative success of spraying operations.   In
the former case an epidemiological study of malariometric indices may be considered
adequate to provide assurance that malaria transmission has been interrupted.
When however the project is planned specifically for obtaining a statistical
evaluation of the efficacy of residual operations, the need for replicating
spraying operations in several groups of villages is desirable.   For this
specific purpose the plan could be altered by first dividing the entire area into
a number of large-sized regions each containing a group of several villages.
Half the number of these large regions will be allocated at random to the sprayed
group and the remainder will be left unsprayed.   For the purpose of evaluation,
a central village may be designated as the observational village in each region
so that within each sprayed region the observational village will be one surrounded
by a sprayed area, thus minimizing the risk of infection being brought over from
the unsprayed areas.   The effect of intermingling of population can of course be
separately studied if parasite rates are calculated separately for such individuals
as could not have moved out (children under three to four years, invalids, etc.).
In any case, supplementary information should be recorded in respect of each new
malaria case to show whether the person had spent some previous nights in the
unsprayed region.

It need hardly be stated that the planning of such a field trial should take
into account the migratory habits of the people, the distances at which individual
villages are situated and other local conditions such as the prevailing species of
mosquitos etc., which determine malaria transmission.

Recent developments in the statistical methodology of designing experiments
have provided several standardized patterns for field work which could well be
adopted in connexion with malaria demonstration.   These standardized designs are
intended to provide the maximum amount of information at the minimum operational
cost.

4.2 Malaria Experimental Pilot Project

The purpose of such a project may be, for instance, to test the relative efficacy of at least three or more different insecticides, namely DDT, BHC and dieldrin, in the control of malaria. It is expected that each of these chemicals may be tried in three or more different ways, thus resulting in nine or more different types of "applications". For the sake of argument let us suppose that we have to study the relative efficacy of nine different "applications". In order to ascertain which of the nine is the best and to evaluate the relative efficacy of each, it is suggested that an area with a sufficiently large number of villages may be selected. If the area has about 100 villages we can try each "application" in about ten villages. The plan visualizes that by the method of random selection (see section 2.20) all the villages in the area will be allocated to the nine different treatments in such a manner that each village receives one "application" and that all the villages receiving any particular type of treatment are distributed randomly over the whole area.

The method of random selection stipulates that a serial list of the total number of villages is first prepared, thus giving each village a serial code number. To these serial numbers will then be allotted at random letters A, B, C, D, E, F, G, H and I, denoting the nine different treatments, as has, for instance, been done in Appendix C. This appendix has been prepared to facilitate the random allocation to cover cases when we may be experimenting with 2, 3, 4, etc. treatments. In the various columns there appear in random sequence as many letters of the alphabet as the number of treatments experimented with. Thus against the serial number of villages shown in the first column there appear in the second column only two letters A and B in random order. If, for example, we were experimenting on ten villages of which five are to be given treatment A and the other five treatment B then this Appendix shows that the first village in our list should receive treatment B, the second and third villages treatment A, the fourth village treatment B, and so forth. As another example, consider the case when we have 90 villages to experiment upon with nine different treatments - each treatment to be replicated over ten villages selected at random. With the help of Appendix C, we could then allocate the nine treatments shown in the last-but-one column against the serial number of the villages (first column).   Thus the first village will get treatment A, the second village C, the third village H and so on.   All the first nine letters of the alphabet thus appear in random order against the serially arranged village code numbers.   By such random allocation we ensure that all the villages receiving treatment A or B etc. are distributed randomly throughout the experimental area, providing us with an estimate on a sample basis, of what the average effect of treatments A, B or C is going to be in that area.   In the use of these lists it is possible that a treatment may appear more frequently than the required number. In that case we should pass over the letters which have appeared the required number of times.

It may be remarked that no provision is being made for keeping certain villages as untreated for purposes of comparison.   The reasons for this are, firstly, that we are primarily interested in determining the relative values of the nine different treatments and, secondly, that to keep some villages untreated may create unpleasant psychological repercussions among the people of the untreated villages.   If it is considered necessary to compare all these different treatments with the experience of untreated villages, the allocation of villages may be made with the help of Appendix C by including an additional letter to indicate the untreated villages.

In this plan it is stipulated that each individual village will constitute a single unit of observation and that for each such population unit, separate malariometric indices such as spleen rate, parasite rate or infant parasite rate will be estimated.   Malaria indices will be recorded for each village before they are given any treatment, such indices being recorded all over the area at almost the same instant of time to ensure comparability.   Thereafter, changes occurring in these indices will be recorded at periodic intervals.

When the experience of all the villages receiving any one type of "application" is studied by means of these malariometric indices, the average change will give us an estimate of what improvement, if any, could be ascribed to that particular "application".   If we are experimenting on nine different treatments we will thus

obtain nine separate values (or ten if untreated villages were also included) for
each malaria index.   For statistical purposes it will be necessary to test
whether or not these nine averages differ significantly from each other.   If they
do differ and the differences are estimable with desired accuracy, then the
experiment could be terminated.   If they do not so differ it may either be
because a sufficiently large experience has not been accumulated to bring out
statistical significance or that there is no appreciable difference between the
nine treatments.   The latter case might well arise because the population of the
various villages has intermingled.   In the former case it will be necessary to
continue observations for a longer period so that statistical significance is
obtained for differences of magnitude of practical interest.   The question of the
adequacy of sample size is discussed in section 5.

An important point to note in this connexion is that since each application
is repeated several times (ten villages for example) we shall get ten different
values of each malariometric index for each application.   No doubt these values
will differ from each other even though they relate to the same application.   The
degree of variation exhibited within each of these sets of ten values provides the
statistician with a valuable measure of variation that is normally expected to
occur from uncontrollable causes.   This degree of variation constitutes as stated
already a yardstick for testing whether the average value of an index for application A differed from the corresponding average value for application B.   In
other words only when the average value of an index obtained from all villages
treated with A differs from the average of all villages treated with B by an amount
statistically greater than the within-variation shown by a series of ten values, is
the difference between A and B to be considered of statistical significance.

The technique of "analysis of variance" referred to in section 2.18 will
enable us to utilize the within-variation in testing the significance of the
difference among the averages relating to different applications.

4.3   Planning of Projects

An important consideration in the carrying out of field projects is that there
can be different ways of planning the projects, of which some may turn out to be

economical, some unnecessarily elaborate; some may lead to clear-cut assessment of the significance of results, while others may perhaps leave the final results ambiguous. As stated already, recent developments in statistical methodology have contributed greatly to the planning of efficient and economical designs. It is therefore emphasized that collaboration with the statistician should be sought at the stage when the work is being planned, so that not only can he assist in drawing up suitable forms and suggest recording procedures for the collection of relevant statistics, but, what is still more important, he can contribute materially in introducing in the design of the project comprehensiveness, efficiency, economy and conclusiveness.

It has been customary in the past for workers of public health to carry out a project without proper statistical consideration and then submit the data to a statistician to assess the significance of the results of the project. The function of the statistician until recently has been to examine the data and to state the extent to which the results claimed by the experimental worker could have arisen even from chance or from other defects in the plan of the project. In this respect a statistician's unpleasant duty has been not infrequently to point out that the results claimed by the project workers were - to use the unhappy term - "not significant" owing perhaps to inadequate size of the experiment or faulty design. When a statistician assesses the results as not being of significance it is sometimes tantamount to a statement that the experiment was almost a failure inasmuch as it failed to provide a clear-cut answer to the questions put to it. The statistician's task is thus reduced to that of carrying out a "post-mortem" examination of the project and to indicate to the project workers what was the cause of the "death" of the experiment. Neither the statistician nor the project worker would feel happy over this. The tendency today, therefore, is for the project worker to consult the statistician right from the commencement, i.e. in connexion with its planning, for advice as to how the project should be conducted, how many villages should be surveyed, what should be the duration of the survey, how the observations should be recorded and what data would in particular be necessary to evaluate the success of the project.

In this document it is not possible to make suggestions regarding suitable planning, but only to make allusion to some of the pitfalls that should be guarded against.

The broad principles involved in drawing up a plan are based on:

(1) A clear statement of the purpose of the project, i.e. the questions to be answered or the hypotheses to be tested should be clearly stated, implying thereby that the types of numerical information to be collected should be specified in advance.

(2) Description of the plan of the experiment. Once a problem has been clearly stated the next step is to specify the procedure for selecting the size, number and the kind of units to be surveyed or experimented upon; selecting also the treatment combinations; deciding on the accuracy needed in measurements; and determining the general conditions under which the survey or test shall be made and the specifications of the experimental design.

(3) An outline of the method of statistical analysis of the data proposed to be collected. The draft describing in detail the proposed statistical methods for the final analysis and interpretation of results should be prepared before the project is started. It is likely that while working through this analysis a decision may have to be made to change the plan because the proposed project would fail to answer the question at least to the desired precision or because the analysis would tend to become too complicated. The outline of the statistical analysis that should follow the termination of the experiment bears intimate relationship with the questions to be asked and the plan of execution. For well-planned and well-executed surveys or experiments the observations secured should provide an unbiased estimate of the various effects of treatments as well as suitable numerical assessments of the uncertainty or variability of these estimates.

It is the outline of the procedure of the statistical analysis that will determine whether the plan provides for adequate controls and for the estimation of experimental errors.

A wholly unscientific tendency which must always be guarded against is that the results appearing to be in conformity with popular beliefs are accepted at their face value, while attempts are made to explain away the results which may appear contradictory.   A sound experimental technique or design must not only give significant confirmation of the points generally believed to be true, but must also provide a conclusive contradiction of theories if they are not according to expectation.

As stated already, through long experience a number of special techniques and designs have now been developed and perfected which can contribute to economy, conclusiveness and comprehensiveness of the results.

Several methods are recommended for increasing the precision of the project results.   The most common one is to increase the size of the area or project by enlarging the number of units or by prolonging its duration.   In modern experimental designs the need for repetition and randomization is emphasized.   It is by repeating or replicating the observations under similar conditions that we attempt an estimate of error from random causes.

The second method is to use refined techniques for the recording of data and for distributing the observations suitably into different groups.   A good deal of care is necessary in the selection of suitable controls, and the random allocation of the available experimental subjects to the experimental and control groups.

The third method is to record supplementary measurements.   The skilful grouping of experimental units also adds to efficiency in design.   Unnecessarily strict selection should, however, be avoided because if only one particular type of experimental area is used it is possible that the results may not be found applicable in general, based as they would be on a selected material.

It is necessary to take supplementary measurements to remove errors arising from such factors as temperature, rainfall, humidity and other uncontrolled sources of variation.   A number of experimental devices have been developed based on the recognition of the fact that it is neither always possible nor necessary to control all the factors likely to produce variation in results other than the ones to be studied.   For instance, it is an impossible task to choose a sufficiently large number of such villages as could all be considered alike in respect of epidemiology of malaria or specifically with regard to the expected response to treatment.   In fact, the fundamental difference in the modern designing of experiments on living beings and the old experimental methods of physics is that while in the latter case only one factor was allowed to vary at a time, the tendency in modern designing is to permit variation to occur due to a large number of known or suspected factors. The experiment or survey is, however, so arranged that the amount of variation produced in results due to each such factor is capable of separate assessment. In fact, one advantage in permitting several factors to vary simultaneously is that the experimental results so obtained provide a wider inductive basis for drawing conclusions which could be regarded as applicable under a variety of circumstances, and a knowledge of the interaction of different factors can also be obtained.

Further, it may be noted that the task of a malaria worker is even more complex than that of a laboratory worker experimenting on living animals, because he has to experiment on human beings, who cannot be kept in a cage or treated like organisms in a test-tube.   To that extent the planning of field trials requires considerable care and experience.   In this case one of the greatest difficulties lies in selecting suitable controls for the purpose of comparing the effect of the treatments.   When testing the effect of a certain prophylactic measure against disease, the greatest difficulty arises in ensuring that due allowance is made for the marked variation among individuals in respect of exposure to infection.   It is necessary, therefore, to study how some of the field trials have been organized by eminent public health statisticians in recent times, and to adopt their techniques, if applicable.   A pilot field study is necessary before the main investigation is planned.   It often reveals unforeseen difficulties and may indicate how to overcome them.

To quote from <u>The Medical Officer</u> (6 January 1951):

"To determine the value of treatments is the most complex and difficult
matter in all medicine, for it must be undertaken without emotion or bias
of any kind and with complete indifference to the subjects under experiment.
Moreover, the subjects for the experiments must be comparable in all
respects.   These conditions can never be fulfilled when man is used, so
we have to be contented with what is available as near as possible to what
is required.   There is a further ethical difficulty; we must not subject
our fellows to anything which is known to be deleterious, nor deprive him
of benefits to which he is entitled, so all evaluations of treatment start
with obstructions and the results are never wholly trustworthy.   But if
we cannot reach perfection we should get as near to it as we can."

A collection of some useful designs and corresponding discussion will be found in
<u>Experimental Designs</u> by Cochran & Cox, (1950).   For a study of the basic principle,
<u>The Design of Experiments</u> by R. A. Fisher (1951), is recommended.

In connexion with the carrying out of field and hospital trials on antimalarials,
the WHO Expert Committee on Malaria at its third session, emphasized the need of
obtaining results which are comparable.   Certain basic principles which should
guide the workers were listed as follows by the WHO Expert Committee (1950b).

"Chemotherapeutic trials

(1)   Trials should be limited to microscopically diagnosed cases of malaria and
results analysed according to species of parasite.

(2)   Chemotherapeutic agents should be administered only by a competent and
responsible member of the investigation staff.

(3)   The number of cases treated should be sufficiently large to allow adequate
appraisal.

(4)   All available evidence should be given as regards history of previous attacks
of malaria or exposure to infection.

(5)   Trials of a new drug should be run against simultaneous tests with a known
drug.

(6)   The effectiveness of the test drug should be measured by the following
criteria:

(a) subsidence of fever below 100°F; recorded in twelve-hour periods after the first dose;

(b) disappearance of parasitaemia; recorded in days after the first dose;

(c) interval between the end of treatment and reappearance of parasites and/or fever. (The follow-up should preferably extend over a period of one year and statement should be given as to whether the subject has been exposed to re-infection.)

(7) The epidemiological features of the area where the malaria cases under trial acquired the infection should be considered, with particular reference to:

(a) endemicity of malaria;

(b) antimosquito measures in force, and with what success;

(c) transmission season;

(d) degree of severity of the malaria season in the investigation period as compared with previous years.

Suppressive treatment trials

(1) The chemotherapeutic agent must be administered only by a competent and responsible member of the investigation staff, who should maintain a register wherein the necessary entry is made against each individual by name at the time the drug is administered.

(2) The population under trial should be as stable as possible and sufficiently large to allow adequate appraisal.

(3) All suspected break-throughs should be confirmed by microscopic diagnosis. They should be treated with the same drug as that used for suppression.

(4) The area selected for trial should be highly endemic or hyperendemic.

(5) The trial of a new drug should preferably be run against simultaneous tests with a known drug in approximately equal groups of persons living in the same locality.

(6) The epidemiological features of the area should be recorded, with particular reference to:

(a) endemicity of malaria;

(b) antimosquito measures in force, and with what success;

(c) transmission season;

(d) degree of severity of the malaria season in the investigation period as compared with previous years."

4.4 Collection and Interpretation of Malaria Statistics and of Related Population, Vital and Health Statistics

If we had a system for the accurate and complete reporting and recording of all cases and deaths from malaria we could, to begin with, tabulate weekly, monthly, or annual figures of malaria attacks and deaths. When these are studied in relation to the size and composition of the population exposed to the risk of malaria, these would not only indicate the magnitude of the malaria problem, but also help in establishing the seasonal incidence, periodic or epidemic cycles over a number of years, any systematic long-term trend towards increase or decrease of malaria, as well as the degree of variation expected from other random factors from time to time.

Unfortunately, malaria cases in the general population are not always notified, nor do all malaria cases receive treatment in hospitals or get seen by doctors. The correct recording of malaria cases is, among other things, also dependent upon the diagnostic facilities available.

In many countries and over large areas of the world, public health services have established a notification system by which reports of cases of certain preventable diseases are promptly made to the health department. The reporting of malaria cases through such notification services as a routine measure, is however, of doubtful value. The information can best be collected by repeated house-to-house visits and not merely by reliance on the voluntary reports of individuals or physicians. Of course, where malaria is prevalent in an endemic form, the people

become familiar with the nature of malaria attacks, from their characteristic
syndrome of chills-fevers-sweats, and commonly regard the disease with indifference,
owing in part to the ready availability of specific medicaments.   Even in well-
developed countries there is reason to believe that a good deal of self-diagnosis
and self-treatment of malaria infections occurs, therefore it becomes difficult
to judge the morbidity level.   As Covell et al. (1953), and Boyd (1949), have
clearly pointed out, malaria morbidity reporting for the general population is
either altogether non-existent or is notoriously incomplete and unreliable, even
in developed countries.   This is because of the very nature of the disease
complicated by the attitudes of both patients and physicians.   As regards patients
for instance, in areas where medication and medical advice is available, there is
no disease where self-diagnosis and self-treatment is indulged in to a greater
extent than is malaria, with relief of symptoms by suppression but not by complete
cure.   While this factor may not be serious in the case of quartan and benign
tertian infections, in the case of primary malignant tertian cases this would
indeed introduce important errors.   Further, malaria especially of the malignant
tertian type, may complicate or be complicated by a host of other diseases.   Consequently, in malarious areas it may be wrong both to regard a malaria-like disease
as malaria only, or not to consider the individual as suffering from malaria at all.
Another complication in connexion with malaria morbidity reporting arises because
of the chronic relapses and frequency of multiple and super-infections.   Furthermore,
after the illness, the parasitaemia may get reduced to submicroscopic proportions
either through the effects of self-medication or from natural causes.   The nature
of the disease further presents difficulties in the definition of a case of malaria,
while the population at risk may be even more difficult to estimate.   One has to
distinguish between primary attacks and various types of relapses, multiple and
super-infections, which give combinations of quotidian, remittent, intermittent and
continuous fevers.   Further, we have to distinguish between indigenous and
imported cases.   Boyd (1949), therefore, suggests that the term "cases" of malaria
should be substituted by the term "attacks" and the latter must be studied with
regard to each clinical episode to distinguish recrudescences from relapses - if
not other types.   For these reasons, he has suggested that if malaria morbidity

reporting is to be utilized for statistical purposes, each individual report should first be studied with reference to date of onset of the illness, diagnosis, place of residence, age, sex, race, etc. as it is under these circumstances only that each report has factual value. Therefore, as already stated, the only method of judging the level of malaria in a community is by house-to-house investigation - a procedure which is both time-consuming and costly: much persuasion may be necessary to get a blood smear. For a proper assessment of the disease considerable patience is required to interrogate the householders and to investigate every clinical episode, as well as to undertake microscopic verifications rather than limit the collection of information to presumptive primary attacks.

In regard to mortality from malaria, in many advanced countries where persons are examined and treated by qualified doctors, systems have been established for the reporting and registering of deaths occurring from different causes. A death certificate is filed by the attending physician in which a statement as to cause of death is made. Not infrequently, however, a death certificate may be filed by a physician who did not see the patient before death; the recorded diagnosis is then based on the account received from the head of the family. Furthermore, in under-developed areas, especially in rural malarious areas, the reporting of both malaria cases and deaths is generally far from complete or accurate. Over large areas malaria deaths may happen to be reported merely as deaths from "fevers". For example, in rural areas of India, which are not yet adequately covered by public health and medical staff, and where the cause of death is made by lay persons, malaria deaths are recorded merely as "fevers" or included in the category "all other causes". In such cases the trend of fever cases or fever deaths from month to month may be the only means of obtaining an idea of the seasonal periodicity of malaria; or, as is explained in section 4.4.3, for judging the relative and absolute trends of malaria. Even in well organized hospitals, unless laboratory aids are resorted to, malaria deaths occurring mostly due to malignant tertian infections and taking cerebral or algid forms, may get confused or missed, especially in the case of patients arriving in a moribund state and dying within a few hours of admission. Of course, in rural areas where neither physicians nor laboratory

services are available, such cases and deaths may be entirely missed.   However,
in the case of regional and fulminating epidemics of malaria, the diagnosis may be
rendered easier on a group scale where large numbers become infected.

The problem is to extract the maximum amount of relevant information from the
available recorded statistics, and to help and initiate action in building up
additional suitable statistical records so as to obtain an increasingly more
reliable picture of the malaria problem.   Among the records which are generally
available even in the relatively less developed areas are figures of malaria cases
treated in hospitals or dispensaries.

4.4.1   Hospital and dispensary statistics

In spite of certain statistical difficulties of interpretation which are
referred to later, the records of admissions from malaria in hospitals and dispensaries constitute a valuable source of information on morbidity from this
disease, because generally these cases are diagnosed by medical personnel.   However,
the popularity of the hospital staff, the availability of transport facilities for
the patients to reach these institutions, the concentration of the people around
the dispensary, the severity of the attacks, the availability of private medical
practitioners, practices of self-medication and self-diagnosis, the economic level
of the people, diagnostic facilities available, are all factors that affect the
numbers of those seeking admissions or recorded as suffering from malaria in
hospital registers.   It is therefore, not possible to relate these figures to any
population as the base for working out malaria morbidity rates, i.e. persons
attacked by malaria per 100 000 population in a specified period, usually a year.
In some cases, attempts have been made to obtain from the local private medical
practitioners the figures of malaria cases treated by them (if they have such
records) and thereby to arrive at a more complete figure.   This total figure,
when divided by the population of the area served by the dispensary, may serve to
provide a rough idea of the malaria morbidity rate, but its use is generally not
to be preferred.   However, in the case of such closed populations as the Army,
gaols, or other institutions, malaria morbidity figures may indicate in a fairly
reliable manner the average incidence, of course only in that selected type of
population.

Even though hospital figures cannot satisfactorily reflect the level of malaria sickness in the community, they are nevertheless useful for the study of certain aspects of the disease, especially the seasonal prevalence, the relationship of malaria incidence to climatic factors, and the degree of variability from year to year over short periods of time. But as has been pointed out by Hill, Cambournac & Simoes (1943) dispensary and hospital statistics often fail to distinguish between relapses and reinfections, as the diagnosis is generally made with respect to the current illness without reference to previous infections. These authors observed infants and children over a period of five years to study the effect of relapses and reinfections on spleen and parasite rates. Sometimes data on malaria sickness are collected by house-to-house visits from interviews with the occupants. This may involve considerable expense and labour, and the response from the people may be satisfactory generally when they are assured that free treatment will be offered to all types of diseases. Such data are highly influenced by the time of the year the visits are made, i.e. before, during or after the period of the epidemic, and on the co-operation that the team can secure from the public. Collection of such data provide as it were a snapshot picture of malaria in the community. The percentage of persons who are found suffering from the disease to the total number of persons examined, provides a measure of the prevalence of the disease in the community.

4.4.2 Recorded health statistics

It has been mentioned already that over large parts of the world and especially in the so-called under-developed areas with endemic malaria, statistical information bearing on the state of health of the people is either unreliable or entirely lacking. No doubt attempts for improvement are being made by respective national governments and by international organizations, especially the Statistical Office of the United Nations and the World Health Organization. Time and again resolutions are passed and specific action suggested for effecting such improvement. Malaria workers will do well, therefore, to study the systems in force for the collection of health statistics instituted by national governments in the areas chosen for field work. As far as possible, instead of setting up a system of their own to

record vital and health statistics, it is hoped that they would collaborate with
the existing staff in improving the quality of statistics collected for the area.
Proper investigation should be made as to the various sources of error or omissions
in the data collected, and facilities available for compilation and analysis.
Advice and assistance rendered to national officials already engaged in operating
the vital statistics registration systems will materially help in developing an
improved system of statistics for the country, and especially for the area in which
malaria workers may be carrying out their investigation or demonstration work.

It is relevant to quote here the recommendation of the Malaria Conference in
Equatorial Africa (WHO 1951b) in regard to biostatistics concerning malaria:

"In the absence of trustworthy and comprehensive data relating to the
effect of malaria on the population, the conference recommends that all
governments should give the matter of biostatistical returns the most
careful attention, so that the development of control of malaria may be
accurately assessed."

From among the figures recorded on a national scale the following types of
vital and health statistical data will be found convenient and meaningful either
to describe properly the health and demographic conditions of the area for public
health and epidemiological purposes, or to provide basic documentation in support
of the results of antimalaria campaigns.   Such information, which as stated
already, is routinely collected, can be obtained for individual localities as well
as for larger population groups.   In any case, it is necessary to distinguish
between information relating to urban or rural characteristics of the area.   In
so far as no internationally agreed definition of urban or rural areas has yet
been put forward because of the difficulties of reconciling differences in the
use of these terms in different countries, it would be appropriate to state clearly
the definitions used.

It is advisable to collect the following data for a number of previous years:

(a) Estimated population of the area at the middle of the year; classified
by age and sex if possible.

(b) Total number of live births.

(c) Total number of deaths classified by major causes of death.

(d) Total number of deaths attributed to malaria. If total deaths from malaria are not available, deaths under the broad heading "fever" may be obtained.

(e) Total number of deaths among children under one year of age, and if possible among children in age-groups 1-4, 5-9 years, etc.

Based on these data the following rates could be calculated for each year:

1. Crude live-birth rate per 1000 population.

2. Death rate from all causes per 1000 population.

3. Malaria death rate per 100 000 population.

4. Infant mortality rate per 1000 live births.

The following numerical examples will illustrate the use of the formulae given above for calculating various rates. Basic data are set out in Table 41 below:

Table 41. Guatemala. Vital statistics data for 1952

Mid-year population	2 975 000
Live births	151 865
Deaths from all causes	71 994
Deaths from malaria	6 947
Deaths among children under 1 year of age	17 036

From these basic data the rates are computed as follows:

1. Birth rate $= \dfrac{151\ 865 \times 1000}{2\ 975\ 000} = 51.0$

2. Death rate from all causes $= \dfrac{71\ 994 \times 1000}{2\ 975\ 000} = 24.2$

3. Malaria death rate $= \dfrac{6\ 947 \times 100\ 000}{2\ 975\ 000} = 233.5$

4. Infant mortality rate $= \dfrac{17\ 036 \times 1000}{151\ 865} = 112.2$

These rates, if collected for each of a number of years prior to the starting of the campaign, will be useful for establishing a report.   But attention should be paid to their reliability and intrinsic meaning in the period under consideration, especially as to how complete they were and are now, and to changes which might have occurred in the way the figures were collected, which might have affected their significance.

4.4.3   Epidemic figure

In those areas where the registration of causes of death is unreliable or where malaria deaths are registered mostly under the heading "fevers", it is not easy to study variation in malaria mortality from the official records.   If the registration of total deaths is satisfactory and malaria recurs in epidemic form, an index called "Epidemic Figure" (Gill, 1928) may be found satisfactory.   It is based on the knowledge that generally malaria epidemics in a locality have a clearly marked seasonal periodicity, as, for instance, following the rains in several areas.   If, therefore, fever deaths reported in the post-rainy months in any year were high, an assumption may be made that malaria was the responsible cause for this increase provided, of course, that some other disease also was not known to have risen to epidemic proportions at the same time, a fact that could generally be verified from hospital or dispensary statistics.   To find out the value of "epidemic figure" the average number of deaths in the three known malarious months should be first calculated.   The average monthly deaths in the previous three non-malarious months are also calculated separately.   For gauging the actual intensity of an epidemic of malaria, the index called the "epidemic figure" may be worked out by dividing the average monthly fever deaths during the three malarial months of the same year by a similar average for the three previous non-malarious months.[1]   The "epidemic figure" thus obtained would indicate the number of times the mean monthly fever mortality during the malaria months exceeded the mean monthly fever mortality in the non-malaria

---

[1] In WHO "Malaria Terminology" (see Covell et al., 1953, page 30) epidemic figure is stated as the number of deaths in a selected epidemic month divided by the normal monthly deaths for the area.   The definition adopted by previous Indian workers is therefore somewhat different from that stated by Covell et al.

period the same year.   In normal years, that is, when the area remains free from
malaria epidemics, the epidemic figure is generally found to be about 1.0.   It
tends to increase in proportion to the increase in malaria mortality, and in years
of epidemics this figure may be found to be as high as 10 in certain localities.
When there is an epidemic of malaria, the epidemic figure for large tracts is
approximately 2.5.   By plotting such epidemic figures on a map for small registration areas, the intensity and distribution of regional epidemics can be studied.
One objection to the use of this figure, as already stated, is that if any other
disease also had a tendency to increase in the same months as malaria, an epidemic
of that disease will also change the epidemic figure.   Again, based as it is only
on figures of deaths, no account is taken of the actual morbidity.   In some malaria
endemic areas it is known that malaria cases may increase without appreciably
increasing the fatality.   The epidemic figure does not therefore reflect the
actual prevalence of the disease in a relatively mild form and fails to provide
a reliable index of malaria prevalence.   In any case, while an increase in the
epidemic figure in an area may indicate the occurrence of an epidemic of malaria,
a low value of this figure may be compatible with the occurrence of an epidemic
of a mild type involving low mortality.   In the absence of any other monthly
figures relating to malaria, the epidemic figure can indicate roughly the long-
term trend of the disease and may be found useful in assessing the results of
control measures.

4.4.4   <u>Spleen rate, parasite rate, etc.</u>

<u>Spleen rate</u>

Enlargement of the spleen is so characteristic of an attack of malaria that
it has long been the practice to use splenic palpation as a means of obtaining
useful indices of the prevalence, distribution and intensity of malaria in a
locality.   Spleen examination has the advantage that it can be carried out rapidly
under field conditions without the use of appliances.   It is usually carried out
on children examined in their homes during a house-to-house survey, or in schools.
Examination of schoolchildren has the further advantage of the availability of a
larger number of children in one place, and the possibility of follow-up examinations

of the same group at different times. An index called the spleen rate is calculated as the percentage of persons showing splenomegaly to the total number of persons examined. The spleen rate based on examination of only the school-going children, relates to a selected sample and is generally lower in value than that for the general child population, possibly owing to the relatively higher social status of schoolchildren, the sick children being absent and the children under five years being unrepresented. In addition, the use of antimalarial drugs administered by school-teachers influences the results as also does the fact that the schoolchildren may be drawn from a wider area, such as from neighbouring villages.

These advantages and disadvantages of basing spleen rates on the examination of schoolchildren alone should be weighed locally, as conditions differ from one area to another. It is also possible, that in an area with a home-associated vector of limited flight range, the spleen rate obtained by taking children from near the breeding place itself may yield a higher spleen rate than for the entire population. In any case, it is necessary to remember that a house-to-house survey on a random sample of village children would yield a statistically acceptable estimate of the spleen rate.

In so far as the spleen rate in children may differ from that in adults, it has been recommended in Malaria Terminology that the spleen rate be calculated as the percentage of children aged 2-9 years showing palpable enlargement of the spleen. This age-group may be further divided into two groups 2-4 years and 5-9 years.

Among other measures based on spleen examination it may suffice to mention the average enlarged spleen. As is explained in Malaria Terminology this index is represented by a number arbitrarily determined. It is essential for purposes of comparison that the standard classification of spleen enlargement recommended in Malaria Terminology and no other, be followed.

In comparing spleen data for different localities or at different times, it is necessary to keep in mind the various factors which are likely to produce variation in results such as for instance the personal bias of the examiner, the procedure adopted for palpation of the spleen (whether the subject is examined standing, sitting, or lying down), the age distribution of the group examined, the time of examination in relation to malaria season, etc. Unless proper allowance is made for these factors the value of the data for the purposes of comparison is vitiated.

The percentage of individuals showing parasites, to the total number of persons examined, gives the parasite rate. If the examination is confined to children aged 0-11 months, the rate obtained is the "infant parasite rate". The age-group 2-9 years is also used in the calculation of parasite rates as both the spleen and blood examinations can be done on the same group of children. The infant parasite rate is of special importance when studying the amount of transmission during the previous year, season of transmission, the seasonal distribution of various plasmodia and when judging the effectiveness of control measures. This is because infants could acquire infection locally having been exposed to infection during one transmission season only. This rate is to some extent dependent on the time devoted to the examination of each slide.

The number of parasites per mm^3 of blood in any given individual is the parasite count. From these individual values two estimates, namely the mean parasite count, or the mean positive parasite count, can be calculated, the former taking into account negative observations also, while for the latter only the value of actual infections is taken. Since the individual figures may show enormous variation, even a single figure of very great magnitude may swamp the effect of a majority of much smaller counts. For this reason, when calculating an average the use of arithmetical mean is not recommended, mode or median being preferred. The use of geometric mean is another method used to allow for extreme deviations.

It is not proposed in this handbook to discuss various other malariometric indices defined and described in Malaria Terminology. Brief comment made above in respect of spleen and parasite data will show that great care should be exercised in the interpretation of such data, paying due attention to the number of individuals on which observations were carried out, the effect of different sources of variation detracting from comparability, such as the time, place, investigator, and technique used and method of selecting the sample for examination.   Further, in the interest of international comparability, the definitions of the terms used should be those set out in Malaria Terminology.

4.5   Interpretation of Vital and Health Statistics Rates in Malaria Work

Generally speaking, in evaluating the effect of the campaign on individual malariometric indices, a comparison with previous trends over the course of several years is to be attempted rather than a comparison with data relating merely to one or two years prior to the campaign.   Other facts which might have influenced their present behaviour outside the action of the antimalaria campaign should not be overlooked.

It has been pointed out by Pampana (1954) that when dealing with figures of malaria morbidity or mortality the rates calculated on national totals may be meaningless if only part of the national territory is malarious.   Thus, malaria death rates in Nicaragua and Madagascar, where the whole national territory has been an endemic area, would convey to us some idea of the importance of malaria as a cause of death.   On the other hand, the malaria death rate for the whole of the United States of America some 40 years ago was extremely low, thus masking the fact that in some States malaria was an important cause of death.   In Tennessee, for instance, the malaria death rate in 1914 was 28.6 per 100 000 population, whereas the malaria death rate for the whole of the United States of America "registration area" was only 2.2.

This consideration is indeed fundamental when we wish to study the success of malaria control measures over a long period of time.   It would then be necessary to calculate annual series of malariometric indices separately for those areas or field stations for which the epidemiology of malaria is known to be different because of topography, climate, species of vector, or the degree of malaria endemicity, etc. It would therefore, first of all, be necessary to divide the entire area into various strata with respect to malaria and to evaluate the indices separately for each stratum.

Another point to be kept in mind, especially in connexion with the countries showing high malaria mortality, is that the figures for both morbidity and mortality for malaria are not sufficiently reliable because of lack of facilities for determining the cause of death or because the system for the registration of malaria deaths may be unsatisfactory. For this reason, it would seem appropriate not only to examine the recorded malaria statistics but also to study variations in the crude death rate, provided the general mortality data are acceptable as regards completeness of registration. Clearly, the higher the malaria mortality the greater will be the proportion of malaria deaths in all deaths, and the greater will be the reduction in the crude death rate after malaria has been controlled. But in a country where, in spite of high malaria morbidity, the mortality from this disease is low, then it would not be legitimate to ascribe any reduction in the general death rate to antimalaria work. In this connexion, Pampana compares the experience of Italy and Ceylon; the former, with high malaria morbidity but low malaria mortality, against the latter with both mortality and morbidity at a high level. In the following Fig. 28 reproduced from his paper, a comparison is made between the trend in the death rates from malaria mortality and the death rate from all causes. In Ceylon, following the application of malaria control measures in 1946, the descent of the crude death rate was more steep than in Italy. The difference between the two countries was more marked as regards the malaria mortality rate, suggesting that the decrease of malaria mortality in Ceylon may well be largely responsible for the decline of the crude death rate in the island, but that in Italy it is relatively much less so. Pampana has studied the experience of other countries, and has expressed doubts as to whether the disappearance of malaria from countries of high malaria mortality could by itself explain decreases in the death rate because it has to be remembered that DDT has gone hand in hand with antibiotics, because insecticidal spraying often controls other insect-borne diseases and also because repeated visits to the families by personnel of the health services might have had health educational value. Furthermore, such other factors as improvement in economic conditions and in environmental sanitation would also have had similar effects.

Fig. 28

CRUDE DEATH RATES AND MALARIA DEATH RATES IN CEYLON AND IN ITALY BEFORE AND AFTER MALARIA CONTROL
(PER 100,000 INHABITANTS)

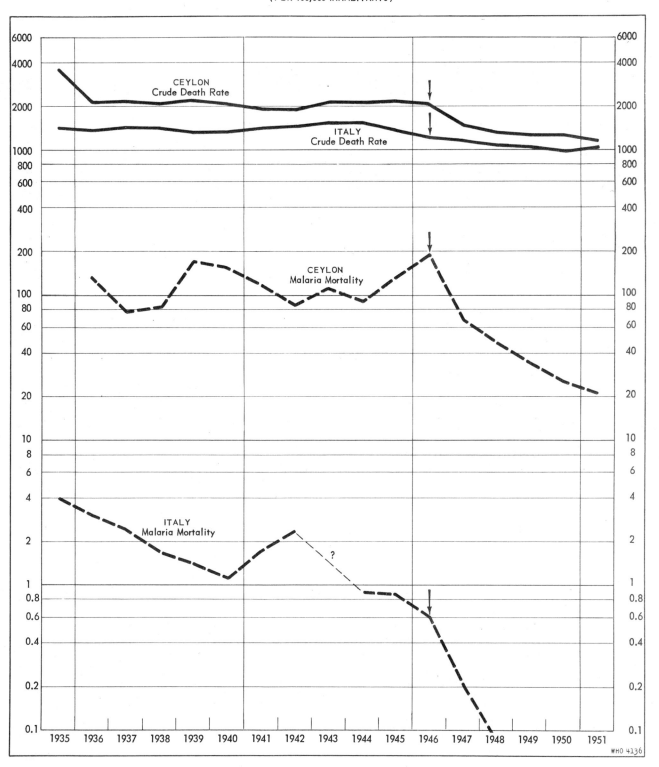

WHO 4136

The above remarks are, of course, applicable to infant mortality rates also, but it is known that the more highly endemic malaria is, the more immunity develops with age, so that malaria tends to become more a children's disease, restricting its victims to the younger ages. For this reason it is to be expected that malaria control in highly endemic countries will bring about a remarkable decrease in infant death rates. This is borne out by the experience in Ceylon in which the decrease in the infant mortality rate has been much more dramatic in malarious districts than in others (Pampana, 1951).

Apart from infant mortality rates, specific death rates at other ages also have considerable interest to a malaria worker. For instance, after a mass antimalaria campaign in an area, it is of interest not only to examine the decrease in the crude death rate or the infant mortality rate, but also in specific death rates at various age-groups (see section 3.3.3). The general experience is that the decrease at various ages is not uniform because persons in the more advanced age-groups, being relatively more immune, would show lesser gains from control of malaria than younger ones in the yet susceptible category. As an example we may quote the experience in Ceylon following the island-wide malaria control campaign by DDT which commenced in the year 1946. In Table 42 the age-specific death rates in the years 1946 and 1954, together with the percentage of 1954 rates to 1946 rates, are given. Relatively higher gains are recorded in the young age-groups 10-44 years; the lowest percentage decrease is for the age-group 65 years and over.

Table 42.   Ceylon.   Decrease in age-specific death rates per thousand between 1946 and 1954

Age	Age specific death rate in		Percentage of (3) to (2)
(1)	1946 (2)	1954 (3)	(4)
Under 5	67.9	36.9	54
5-9	7.0	3.6	51
10-14	3.4	1.3	38
15-19	5.1	1.4	27
20-24	8.6	2.6	30
25-34	9.9	3.3	33
35-44	12.0	4.3	36
45-54	17.2	7.4	43
55-64	29.6	15.7	53
65 and over	98.9	74.7	76

Figures in respect of birth rates also have relevance in connexion with the study of malaria because the disease may lead to an interruption of pregnancy, which may in part be explained by the various types of anaemia that it causes and in part by the well-known predilection of malaria parasites, in particular P. falciparum for the placenta. The following diagram (Fig. 29) showing the variation in annual births and deaths registered in Madagascar, 1934-54, indicates that with the start of the island-wide antimalaria campaign in 1949 annual births began to increase while annual deaths registered a slight decline (G. Joncour, 1956).

It is to be noted, however, that although it may appear logical therefore that malaria may to some extent reduce the number of live births, the available data on the influence of malaria on birth rates may sometimes be contradictory. This study is complicated by the fact that following a malaria campaign the registration of births or of deaths of infants within the first few months of life which previously were not recorded, may happen to be recorded to an increasing degree, and therefore show not only an apparent increase in the birth rate but also a corresponding apparent decrease in the death rate. The extent to which improved registration of births or erroneous calculation of basic population estimates can affect the conclusion, should be carefully investigated.

It need hardly be emphasized that when individuals are examined for spleen enlargement or for the presence of malaria parasites in the blood, no reliable conclusions are possible unless the total number of persons examined (i.e. with and without spleen enlargement or with and without malaria parasites) is also taken into account. As an interesting illustration of the fallacy that can arise without this precaution we may consider the following hypothetical data relating to blood examination of 20 146 persons carried out in a community, of whom 2879 were found to be positive for malaria parasites. The results expressed in five-year age-groups are shown in Table 43:

Fig. 29 Madagascar. Births and deaths 1934-1954

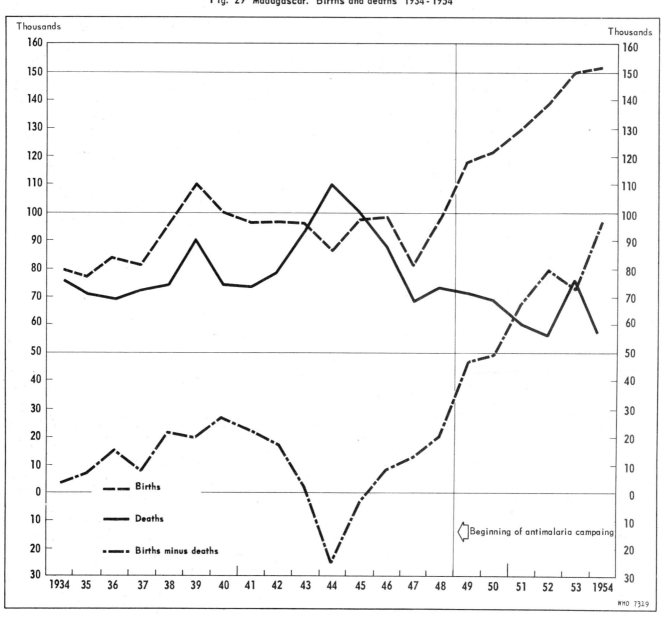

Table 43.   Age distribution of persons found positive for
malaria parasites

Age	Persons
0 - 4 years	580
5 - 9	1 054
10 - 14	510
15 - 19	225
20 - 24	145
25 - 29	90
30 - 34	46
35 - 39	41
40 - 44	41
45 - 49	20
50 - 54	28
55 - 59	25
60 years and over	74
All ages	2 879

It is seen from this table that the number of persons found positive is the largest
in the age-group 5-9 years and the numbers decrease rapidly with advancing age (see
also Fig. 30).   This may lead one to conclude that the immunity of the population
to malaria was low at the earlier ages and that it increased rapidly with age.   But
if we remember that the number found positive depends not only on the degree of
malaria infection but also on the total number examined in each age-group, such a
conclusion would be unacceptable unless the number examined was the same at all
ages - which is not the case as shown by column 2 of Table 44.

Table 44.   Age distribution of persons examined and found
positive for malaria parasites

Age	Persons examined	Persons found positive	Percentage positive
(1)	(2)	(3)	(4)
0 - 4 yrs	3 476	580	16.7
5 - 9	6 982	1 054	15.1
10 - 14	4 013	510	12.7
15 - 19	1 314	225	17.1
20 - 24	756	145	19.2
25 - 29	615	90	14.6
30 - 34	409	46	11.2
35 - 39	402	41	10.2
40 - 44	515	41	8.0
45 - 49	213	20	9.4
50 - 54	372	28	7.5
55 - 59	294	25	8.5
60 yrs and over	785	74	9.4
All ages	20 146	2 879	

When the total number of persons examined differs from one age group to another,
a suitable measure to be used is the age specific parasite rate, i.e. the percentage
of persons found positive for each age group.   In the above table the last column
shows age-specific parasite rates.   These percentages are plotted in Fig. 31 which
yields a different pattern from the one obtained by an examination of merely the
number of positive persons.   The peak has now shifted from the age-group 5-9
years to 20-24 years and the decrease thereafter is not so well marked as in the
previous case.   Interesting examples of variation in immunity and infection by
age are provided by Schuffner (1938).

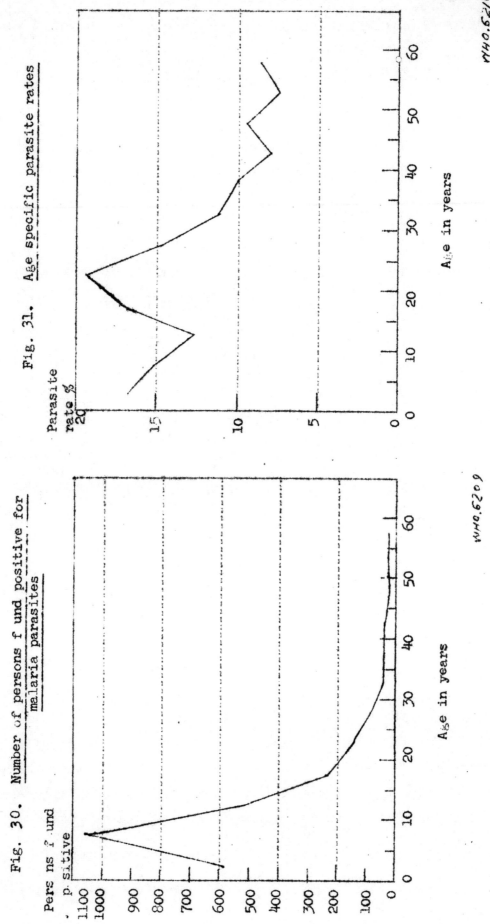

Fig. 30. Number of persons found positive for malaria parasites

Fig. 31. Age specific parasite rates

4.6   Assessment or Evaluation of Malaria Projects

Undoubtedly malaria imposes significant physical, economic and social burdens
on individuals, communities and nations.   It is therefore logical to expect that
after a significant reduction has been produced in malaria incidence or mortality
in an area, there should be an improvement not only in the health of the people but
also in their social and economic well-being.   Governments or other agencies
concerned with malaria projects naturally wish to study the cost of malaria control
or eradication in relation to the losses the disease causes.   Therefore the
measurement of the economic and social effects assumes importance.   But how can
such benefits be objectively assessed and brought into focus?

The Second Asian Malaria Conference at Baguio, Philippines in 1954 (WHO, 1956a)
listed the following among the benefits commonly attributed to successful malaria
control projects:

(a) Lower infant and general mortality rates.

(b) Reduced absenteeism among schoolchildren, public servants, and
workers in general.

(c) Reduced incidence of certain insect-borne diseases such as
plague, leishmaniasis, filariasis, and certain intestinal infections.

(d) Increased and more uniform use of land.

(e) Increased tourism.

(f) Increased public understanding of, and co-operation in public
health and welfare programmes.

These are in addition to preventing losses from malaria as listed below:

A.   Losses due to malaria illness

(1) Earnings forfeited because of physical incapacity, time spent
nursing others, and repayment of unusual debts, cost of medical care
(quacks, physicians, hospitals, medicines), cost of spiritual care
(priests, candles, sacrifices).

(2) Lessened efficiency while chronically ill or convalescent,
resulting in lower output of labour, smaller or fewer crops, lack
of energy to plan effectively or to obtain a better job.

B. **Losses due to malaria deaths**

Value of a life lost.

C. Losses due to malaria endemicity, such as lower rentals, depreciated real
estate, forced sales, moving from endemic areas, difficulty or impossibility of
utilizing or reclaiming land for resettlement, cultivation, or other developments,
and increased costs of public works such as roads and irrigation projects.

While many of these gains and losses may be numerically measured, it is not
unlikely that the presence of other debilitating uncontrolled diseases such as
hookworm or bilharziasis, may still continue to undermine the health of the people.
Further, increased agricultural or industrial production would also depend on the
availability of facilities for work to the people of the area.   Therefore, even
though agricultural or industrial production may logically be expected to increase
through an improvement in the malaria situation, if such an improvement is not
discernible it should not be argued that malaria control did not bring about health
benefits to the people.   It would also be a mistake to compare production in the
year or few years immediately following malaria control measures with that in the
pre-operational years, for it may happen that for other reasons these years may
otherwise have been very good or very bad for agricultural produce.   This is
because of the well-known fact that agricultural harvest is considerably affected
by meteorological factors or availability of water at the opportune time, etc.,
failure of which may have devastating effects.   Further, considerable differences
are known to arise in the evaluation of an agricultural yield of an area by the
adoption of different methods of estimation.   In the more developed countries of
the world, where highly objective and scientific methods of crop cutting experi-
mentation are used to assess crop yield, reliable estimates are prepared.
Unfortunately, areas highly endemic for malaria are also generally the so-called
under-developed ones where such scientific and reliable methods of crop estimation

may neither be in use nor may trained staff be available to employ them. Under
such circumstances, crop yield may happen to be judged only subjectively i.e. based
on the opinions of individuals rather than on measurements, and may therefore be a
highly unreliable and statistically unsound index of agricultural yield. Similar
arguments generally apply to the assessment of economic level of the people.

In view of these considerations it may not be altogether advantageous or easy
to appraise the beneficial effects of malaria control through such indirect measures
as improvement in economic, social, or agricultural prosperity, as a number of other
facts may tend to produce variability in such conditions. If, however, it is considered essential that such effects be judged, it is suggested that the judgement
be based not on figures of one or two years, but on the recorded experience of a
longer series of years, and that the help of scientists versed in the assessment of
agricultural production or economic conditions should be sought, and not left either
to the local lay people or untrained government officials.

An interesting study of economic and social effects of malaria control with
some specific instances from Taiwan has been provided by Pletsch & Ch'en (1954).

In the recent past WHO has been engaged in developing suitable methodology for
the purpose of project evaluation. Already certain principles for this purpose
have been formulated. (See A. Macchiavello, 1955)

The term "evaluation" has been used by WHO to describe the administrative and
technical procedures by which the value of planned activities are measured for the
benefit of those responsible for their control. As applied to WHO projects it
therefore consists of effectual reporting and assessment of progress made towards
attaining the objectives set out in the plan of operation. The evaluation follows
in its general lines the framework established for this purpose which, briefly
stated, should begin with a brief description of the project for purposes of
identification, followed by a narrative arranged under the following main headings:

     I.   Project area

    II.   Purposes or objectives

   III.   Methods

    IV.   Accomplishments

    V.   Comparative summary

   VI.   Predictions

It is emphasized that project evaluation is a procedure applicable to all the stages of development of the project. Indeed it starts in the planning phase itself as an assessment of the problem - the needs and the resources - as an appraisal of methods and procedures most suitable to their utilization in operations, and as a pre-evaluation or prediction of the expected results. In its wider sense, project evaluation is continued during the whole duration of the project, to assess the efforts and their influence in developing the strategy in achieving the final aims, to condition the timing and phasing of the activities, and to control operations and modify them when a redefinition or a change in direction becomes advisable. Further it is intended not only to evaluate terminal achievements of the project but also to predict the trend and scope of the long-range activities to be developed later so as to help in future planning of other projects through accumulated experience and in decisions concerning further advance in action and better co-ordination in future problems.

Viewed in such a broad perspective the role of statistical methodology would appear to be of a limited scope. Of course, to measure changes, statistics are required before the commencement of the project against which the quality of the accomplishment may be measured. In under-developed areas, however, such statistics of standards may not be available and we may be forced to accept in some cases a subjective appraisal which should be conditioned by and limited to the critical analysis and comparisons of accomplishments against sharply and clearly defined objectives.

4.7 Eradication of Malaria

The Eighth World Health Assembly considered that the ultimate goal of malaria control programmes should be the eradication of the disease. This question is linked up with the potential danger felt in recent years regarding the development of resistance to insecticides in anopheline vector species. The administrative and epidemiological problems involved in malaria eradication programmes have been discussed by Pampana (1955), Macdonald (1956) and Gabaldon (1956), and reported upon by the WHO Expert Committee on Malaria (WHO, 1956b). This section deals with some of the statistical considerations concerning this problem.

The term "malaria eradication" is to be regarded as different from "vector eradication", the latter term implying complete extirpation of the malaria carrying species of anophelines.   "Malaria eradication" on the other hand, "means the ending of the transmission of malaria and of the reservoir of infective cases in a campaign limited in time, carried to such a degree of perfection that when it comes to an end there is no resumption of transmission" (WHO, 1956b).   The plan envisages that no area should be exposed to residual insecticides for more than six years and that neighbouring countries should co-ordinate their programmes so that the cleared country will not be threatened by one where malaria is still endemic.

4.7.1   Criteria of malaria eradication

The evaluation of malaria eradication programmes is based on the following criteria listed by the WHO Expert Committee on Malaria (WHO, 1956b).

Malaria eradication may be assumed when an adequate surveillance system has not discovered any evidence of transmission or residual endemicity despite careful search for three years, in at least the last two of which no specific general measures of anopheline control have been practised.   To establish the claim there should be, in relation to a specific defined area:

(1)   proof that an adequate surveillance system has existed in the area for at least three years, in at least two of which no specific anopheline control measures had been carried out.   Any claim based on a lesser period of post-operational surveillance would need to be supported by proof of a surveillance mechanism above the usual quality;

(2)   evidence that in this period of three years, no indigenous cases, originating within that time, have been discovered;

(3)   the evidence of a register of malaria infections discovered during that time, it being established beyond reasonable doubt that each case was either:

(a)   imported, as shown by the tracing of the case to its origin in an acknowledged malarious area, or

(b) a relapse of a pre-existing infection, as shown by the history of
the case, and the absence of any associated cases in the neighbourhood
of its origin, or

(c) induced, as shown by its relation to a blood transfusion within
an appropriate interval, or to another form of parenteral inoculation
to which infection could be properly attributed, or

(d) directly secondary to a known imported case.

4.7.2 Basic considerations involved

Both Macdonald (1956) and Gabaldon (1956) have rightly pointed out that the
facility with which malaria transmission can be interrupted depends upon several
factors, a prior understanding of which, in relation to the area of operation, is
necessary.   The causes of an outbreak of malaria lie in a source of infection, a
suitable temperature for the development of the plasmodia in the mosquito, and an
anopheline community which is adapted to transmission in its susceptibility, biting
habits, longevity and numbers.   Macdonald (1956) has attempted to summarize the
relative importance of these factors mathematically into a single index termed by
him "the reproduction rate", which in non-mathematical terms is "the number of
infections distributed in a community as the direct result of the presence in it
of a single primary non-immune case".   Even though a precise estimation of the
malaria reproduction rate may be difficult or impossible, he believes that the
general order of magnitude of this rate needs to be understood because in nature
it may vary between one or two and some very large figure such as 5000.   The length
of time taken to reach eradication will depend on the original value of the rate and
the speed of its decrease.   Apart from requiring understanding of the disease in
terms of the malaria reproduction rate, Macdonald's work also emphasizes the very
important role that some undiscovered foci of the disease or some remaining carriers
may play in its future transmission.   The object of an eradication programme,
therefore, is also to discover and eliminate the foci of transmission, to recognize
remaining carriers or incipient epidemics arising from them, and to appreciate the
proper order of events, particularly the expected timing of epidemics arising from
a slow origin.

Gabaldon (1956) has also placed similar emphasis on a prior assessment of what he has termed "the constitution of malaria", described by him in terms of quantity of disease presence as well as its variability under natural circumstances. The quantity of the disease represents as it were its endemicity while the degree of variability from time to time is a sign of its epidemicity. If spleen rates have been estimated for several consecutive years in the locality during the same season, then both these aspects of malaria constitution can be studied in numerical terms. Gabaldon suggests the use of the following two ratios:

Ratio of endemicity: the lowest spleen rate recorded during a period of five to seven years divided by 5 (the figure according to the author corresponds to the normal spleen index, i.e. not due to malaria). The resulting quotient, called the ratio of endemicity is a measure of the minimum prevalence of the disease.

The figure 5 used by the author may vary with age, place and other characteristics. The ratio of endemicity may also vary accordingly.

Ratio of epidemicity: the largest spleen rate recorded in five to seven years (depending on the periodicity of the disease in the area) divided by the smallest.

Areas with frequent transmission throughout the year are characterized by permanently large spleen rates and have a high ratio of endemicity and a low ratio of epidemicity. An area where transmission varies from year to year would have a low ratio of endemicity and a high ratio of epidemicity.

In a locality with low ratios of endemicity and epidemicity with relatively few infected vectors, one application of the insecticide may suffice to stop transmission almost entirely, while in a highly endemic locality some infected vectors may survive and transmission may continue at a low level.

4.7.3   Delineation of endemic foci

It is clear from the foregoing discussion that for the success of the eradication programme a knowledge of the endemic foci of the disease is of great importance. When an area as large as a whole country is to be brought under an eradication plan, the need for detecting as precisely as possible the existence of

such foci is all the more emphasized.   Every bit of information available should be
studied and utilized in carrying out such a search.   More importantly, such data
on disease as are available on a national scale, i.e., from all parts of the country
for a considerable number of preceding years, would be the most valuable.   In
countries where malaria control organizations may have existed for several years,
it may be possible to compile spleen rate figures for a large number of localities
covering practically the whole country.   Gabaldon's ratio of endemicity could then
be worked out separately for each area.   Thus the regions where this ratio is found
to be high can be located.   But for many countries planning eradication programmes
it is improbable that spleen rate data would be available for a long enough period
to indicate conditions throughout the country.   In that case, use could profitably
be made of the available vital statistical information, howsoever imperfect,
especially death rate from malaria by individual localities.   A simple index of
endemicity could first be established for each individual locality as follows.   For
each locality, calculate the annual malaria death rates per 100 000 population for
the last 15 years.   Out of these 15 values, pick out the lowest five and find their
arithmetical mean.   If this average figure is zero or negligibly small, it indicates
that even though the area may have had epidemics of malaria, the conditions are such
as not to maintain the disease at a high level throughout the period studied.   On
the other hand, if this average of malaria endemicity index is found to be relatively
high, it indicates that the disease has had a tendency to persist at a high level,
even in inter-epidemic years or even though there may have been no epidemics.   The
high values of this index are therefore indicative of the existence of malaria
endemic foci.   The geographical distribution of the endemicity index can conveniently be studied on a map, as has been done by way of illustration in Fig. 32 for
Mexico.   The endemicity index of each individual state of Mexico was calculated by
averaging the lowest five malaria mortality rates recorded during the period 1940-
1954.   This map serves at once to pinpoint the areas where the disease has a
tendency to remain in an endemic form.   These are shown to lie in the southern part
of the country.   If morbidity data are available for a long enough period, a similar
map could be constructed by calculating endemicity indices based on malaria morbidity

Fig. 32 Mexico. Malaria endemicity death rate by State, 1940-54

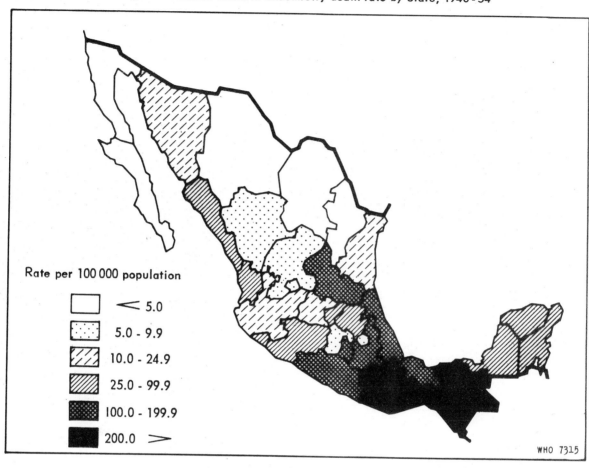

Rate per 100 000 population

☐	< 5.0
⣿	5.0 - 9.9
⫽	10.0 - 24.9
⫽	25.0 - 99.9
⣿	100.0 - 199.9
■	200.0 >

WHO 7315

rates instead of mortality rates.   Similarly, if spleen rate data are available
for a series of years, an average based on the five lowest spleen rates could also
be used to detect malaria endemic foci.

But for many countries with poor registration of causes of death, the deaths
from malaria may not be available on a national scale.   In such countries it may
be advantageous to calculate similar endemicity indices based on all deaths which
fall in the broad group in which malaria deaths are included.   For instance, in
countries where malaria deaths are combined with other deaths from fevers, the
annual death rates from fevers could be studied for a series of 15 years.   Better
results would no doubt be obtained if for each year the fever deaths were considered
only for those two or three months of each year which are known to correspond to
the malaria season.

Once the regions of high malaria endemicity have thus been located, it may
be possible to calculate similar indices for further subdivisions of each of these
units to recognize with greater precision the endemic foci.   For instance, if for
the three states of Mexico showing high endemicity rates, malaria can be tabulated
separately for individual administrative subdivisions of each state, a more
detailed analysis of endemic foci could have been made.   This method of searching
for endemic foci by examining by stages figures for smaller and smaller population
groups has proved valuable in the case of other diseases (Swaroop, 1957) and may
well be applied to malaria.

It is of course understood that malaria eradication programmes, while no
doubt covering all malarious parts of the country, will specially be aimed at the
eradication of the disease from the endemic foci.   Nevertheless, due to administrative
difficulties or errors, some undiscovered small foci may remain from which transmission
may continue.   For this reason, a different technique of approach is needed to detect
and wipe out the residual foci, which may finally prove to be hamlets that were overlooked, or inadequately treated, or lying in inaccessible places, or in places considered non-malarious.

4.7.4 Adequacy of surveillance

According to the WHO Expert Committee on Malaria, eradication can be claimed if an adequate surveillance system has existed in the country for at least three years, and no indigenous case has originated during that time.   How is the adequacy of the surveillance to be judged?

On purely statistical considerations, if we wish to be 95 per cent. sure that no single case in a large-sized population is missed, it would be necessary to take a sample as large as 95 per cent. of the whole population!   This virtually means keeping the entire population under surveillance.   The task is of course believed to be facilitated by the consideration that the aim of surveillance is primarily to discover all cases of fever and to carry out the blood examination only on them. It should be pointed out that this requisite of 95 per cent. coverage of population is not necessarily satisfied if the 5 per cent. are excluded from the sample not on a random basis but because surveillance teams failed to contact them because they were inaccessible or were migrant population.   In this case the 5 per cent. could be biased and may represent a population harbouring the disease.   In actual practice, of course, it would be difficult to ensure that all individuals with past history of fever are contacted.   There is in addition, the possibility that some persons harbouring parasites in the blood may not give history of fever either because of forgetfulness or because of tolerance to parasites.   On these two accounts the observed parasite rate would fall short of the true rate.   If the number of fever cases missed or of subclinical cases of parasitaemia is relatively large, the observed parasite rate may only be a fraction (about half, or even less) of the true rate.   This point should be borne in mind when seeking an assurance regarding the success of eradication.

In areas where the malaria reproduction rate has been known to be low, such a strict surveillance may not be altogether necessary.   Indeed, as has been noted by the WHO Expert Committee on Malaria, "The recognition of absolute freedom from transmission, or of absolute absence of remaining infections, presents insuperable obstacles.   The practical elimination of the vast majority of infections occurs several years before the last one disappears, but experience shows that these last few cases need not in fact re-establish endemicity." For a more practical approach, therefore, if in a large population we are prepared to tolerate the presence of one or two or any other number as the maximum permissible number of cases, the following table will help to indicate the percentage of the total population that should be covered by the surveillance system. For example, if we stipulate that the occurrence of a single case in a large-sized population is tolerated but that we should be able to detect the existence of more than one case with 95 per cent. probability of success, then the table shows that 78 per cent. of the population should be covered, there being of course no biased selection of this sample, i.e. the 22 per cent. of the population not surveyed should in no way be different from the 78 per cent. population brought under surveillance. Stated differently, if there are two cases in the population and if we take a random sample of 78 per cent. of the population, there is a probability of only 5 per cent. that not a single case will be detected in the sample. In other words, when no cases are detected in a sample of 78 per cent. we can safely state that there are no more than two cases in the population; such a statement being true with 95 per cent. probability. A 45 per cent. coverage of the population will ensure that the existence of 5 or more cases is detected with 95 per cent. success but if the number of cases is 4 or less the probability of detecting them with this population coverage is lower than 95 per cent.

Table 45.   Adequacy of the population coverage by surveillance
to detect cases of malaria

Minimum number of cases to be detected with 95% probability	Sample size as percentage of the total population size
1	95
2	78
3	63
4	53
5	45
6	39
7	35
8	31
9	28
10	26

The above table can be used both in cases where we are interested in detecting "fever" cases or only in malaria cases.

In drawing an unbiased sample it is of course not necessary to examine all villages. An unbiased sample can be obtained by multistage sampling, i.e. by first choosing a sample of villages and then examining a sub-sample of the population of only those villages which are included in the first-stage sample of villages. The sample size shown in Table 45 indicates the total percentage of population thus to be examined. Of course when this percentage is very large, a two-stage sampling may be out of the question.

4.7.5 Study of the parasite rate and the spleen rate

No surveillance organization could possibly keep the entire population of the country under a constant watch. All it could possibly do would be to pay periodic visits to various localities. Even if no case of fever is found at the time of the survey, it is likely that a small-scale malaria epidemic may have broken out and subsided prior to the visit of the surveillance unit. In that case, the history of any malaria outbreak, especially of small magnitude, could be studied either by an examination of an adequate number of blood samples or, if considered desirable, by means of the spleen rate. In the case of blood samples, the ideal of course is that the parasite rate should be zero. To ensure that this is so it would be necessary to examine the entire population or the group of the population at risk for which we wish the parasite rate to be zero. The examination of only a sample of the whole population could therefore provide us with an assurance less than certainty that the parasite rate was zero, if no parasites are found in the blood of the population examined. This problem may also be approached in a different way. We may like to be 95 per cent. certain that the parasite rate is at the most 0.1 per cent. in the population. If the limit of the parasite rate is fixed at 0.1 per cent. then, on statistical considerations, it is found that if an unbiased sample of 3000 individuals examined shows no parasite in the blood or even a single one, then this will ensure that the parasite rate was not in excess of 0.1 per cent. On similar considerations we can also say that an examination of 600 individuals - with none showing a parasite in the blood - will ensure (95 per cent. certainty) that the parasite rate in the population was not in excess of 0.5 per cent. These examples are given under the assumption that we are dealing with a large population. If the total number of persons in the area is limited, the sample size required is correspondingly lower. For instance, if the total number of individuals available for examination is 5000, the sample size required for 0.1 per cent. and 0.5 per cent. are about 2250 and 565 respectively. If the population size is about 1000 the corresponding sample sizes are 950 and 450 respectively.

If the malariologist wishes to investigate any possible increase in the spleen rate as a criterion of malaria outbreak then again the sample of children to be examined should be large enough to detect a spleen rate of a stipulated amount, as for instance 5 per cent. or more in the child population. More specifically, we may enquire as to what the sample size should be, so that if no child in the sample showed an enlarged spleen, we could conclude that the spleen rate in the population did not exceed a stipulated limit of 5 per cent. or more. The surveillance should be adequate enough to detect any excess in the spleen rate over this figure. The adequacy of sample size for this purpose has been discussed in a different context in Section 5.5. Use can be made of Table 51 to ascertain how many children should be examined in each locality so that even if one child among them had an enlarged spleen we would say that the spleen rate in the general population in all probability could not be regarded as lower than 5 per cent. This number is around 60 children. If, on the other hand, we are stringent in our demand and ask that the spleen rate should be 1 per cent. or lower in the general population, then about 300 children should be examined in each case, and none should be found to have an enlarged spleen. The sample size indicated here relates to the total population examined and not merely to fever cases in a population of that size.

It may be explained that this sample size is not adequate to determine the rate with any precision. It merely provides us with a test as to whether or not the rate is under 1 per cent. (or 5 per cent.) in the population. For the purpose of estimating the spleen rate with a desired precision, the method of calculating confidence limits should be utilized. Procedures to obtain the adequate sample size for this purpose, are explained in Section 5.4.

4.7.6 Study of the gametocyte carrier

For the detection of gametocytes in the blood, one or more thick film slides are prepared for each person. In this connexion, a question that arises for statistical consideration is how many slides or how many microscopic fields in all should be examined in order to detect the presence of gametocytes in the blood.

It is recognized that however carefully the laboratory worker may prepare different slides for a single individual, the thickness of the blood film will show variation from one slide to another. While in the following discussion we merely estimate the total number of microscopic fields to be examined per individual, it is presumed that such an examination will be spread over several slides from the same person. Of course it is obvious that if the gametocyte density in the blood is high, then examination of only a few fields may reveal the presence of gametocytes. On the other hand, if we are interested in detecting the presence of gametocytes of a low order of density, examination of several fields from different slides would be necessary. Table 46 gives the minimum number of microscopic fields which should be examined to achieve a reasonable degree of assurance that the presence of gametocytes is detected. The theoretical calculations are made on the basis of the minimum total quantity of blood necessary for examination for this purpose. Then, on the assumption that with the technique routinely adopted 0.2 cu. mm of blood was contained in 100 microscopic fields, the minimum number of fields to be examined is estimated. It is possible that owing to variability from one slide to another, 100 fields on a single slide may not correspond to 0.2 cu. mm of blood. But if about 10 different slides are prepared for the same individual by a uniform technique which is intended to ensure 0.2 cu. mm of blood per 100 fields, the average from 10 slides may well approach this standard. Nevertheless, to cover the possibility of variability, Table 46 shows separately the minimum number of microscopic fields required to be examined corresponding to three different cases, namely, when the quantity of blood in 100 fields is on the average either 0.1, 0.2 or 0.3 cu. mm.

The term "reasonable degree of assurance" used earlier means that we wish to be 95 per cent. sure of detection.   Another possibility is that we may wish to be 99 per cent. sure of not missing a gametocyte in the examination.   Table 46 supplies figures corresponding to both these probability levels.

Table 46.   Total number of fields to be examined for 95% or 99% probability of success when the blood film contains 0.1, 0.2 or 0.3 cu. mm of blood per microscopic field

Probable gametocyte density per cu. mm of blood	Film thickness corresponding to blood per 100 fields of:					
	0.1 cu. mm		0.2 cu. mm		0.3 cu. mm	
	probability level		probability level		probability level	
	95%	99%	95%	99%	95%	99%
1	3 000	4 600	1 500	2 300	1 000	1 534
2	2 000	2 300	1 000	1 150	500	767
3	1 000	1 534	500	767	334	512
4	750	1 150	375	575	250	384
5	600	920	300	460	200	307
6	500	767	250	384	167	256
7	429	658	215	329	143	220
8	375	575	188	288	125	192
9	334	512	167	256	112	171
10	300	460	150	230	100	154
11	273	419	137	210	91	140
12	250	384	125	192	84	128
13	231	354	116	177	77	118
14	215	329	108	165	72	110
15	200	307	100	154	67	103
16	188	288	94	144	63	96
17	177	271	89	136	59	91
18	167	256	84	128	56	86
19	158	243	79	122	53	81
20	150	230	75	115	50	77

As an example, let us say that we want to be 95 per cent. sure of being able to detect a gametocyte density of 1 per cu. mm in the case when by the laboratory technique adopted, 100 fields correspond to 0.2 cu. mm of blood.   This table shows that we should examine 1500 fields or 150 fields on each of 10 slides.   Of course, it is possible that a gametocyte may be discovered without having to go through so many fields.   But it is only when an examination of 1500 fields has failed to show the presence of a gametocyte that we can argue that the density was below 1 per cu. mm. As another example, if we want to detect gametocyte density of 5 per cu. mm with the same laboratory technique, this table shows that we should examine 300 fields, which may be spread over three different slides.

One may also ask how great is the probability of detection of a gametocyte when the density is 1, 2, ..., per cu. mm if only 100 fields or 200 fields, etc., were to be examined.   The answer is provided by Table 47 in which the probability percentage of detection for various gametocyte levels has been set out corresponding to the cases when we examine 100, 200, 300, 400 or 500 fields.   This table corresponds to the case when 100 fields contain 0.2 cu. mm of blood.   Reference to the second column of this table will show that if we examine only 100 fields, there is only about 55 per cent. chance that we will detect gametocytes when the density is 4 per cu. mm.

Table 47. The probability (percentage) of detection of gametocytes
corresponding to various field examinations

Probable gametocyte density per cu. mm	Number of fields examined				
	100	200	300	400	500
1	18	33	45	55	63
2	33	55	70	80	86
3	45	70	83	91	95
4	55	80	91	96	98
5	63	86	95	98	99
6	70	91	97	99	99*
7	75	94	99	99*	99*
8	80	96	99	99*	99*
9	83	97	99*	99*	99*
10	86	98	99*	99*	99*
11	89	99	99*	99*	99*
12	91	99	99*	99*	99*
13	93	99	99*	99*	99*
14	94	99*	99*	99*	99*
15	95	99*	99*	99*	99*
16	96	99*	99*	99*	99*
17	97	99*	99*	99*	99*
18	97	99*	99*	99*	99*
19	98	99*	99*	99*	99*
20	98	99*	99*	99*	99*

* This sign indicates that the probability is 99.5% or greater, i.e. well approaching certainty.

5. ADEQUACY OF SAMPLE SIZE

5.1 Introduction

The problem of comparing the effect of any newly discovered drug or vaccine with either the ones already in use or with untreated individuals by means of controlled trials often arises. Whether these trials are carried out on laboratory animals or on human subjects, considerations of cost and time sometimes make it imperative that the number of subjects tested should not be unduly large and yet be large enough to bring out significant differences if they exist. In this connexion, the statistician is frequently asked how many subjects, patients, laboratory animals, etc., should be taken, i.e. how large should the sample be to ensure statistical acceptability of the results.

It should be gratifying to malaria workers to know that the credit for pioneering work done in the preparation of ready-reckoning tables for judging the required size of sample belongs to the eminent malariologist Sir Ronald Ross who, in collaboration with Walter Stott (Ross & Stott, 1911) published as early as 1911, tables of statistical error "specially constructed for practical use in sanitary, pathological and clinical work".

Since the publication of these tables a good deal of literature has appeared on this subject, relating to different types of experiments. The literature is, however, scattered in various scientific journals, many dealing with mathematical theory and as such may be rather inaccessible to malaria workers or may appear couched in a terminology not easy to grasp. It is indeed a difficult task to survey the entire literature on this subject. Nor should it be necessary to do so in view of the fact that many difficult or complex types of experiments would in any case require special treatment. In such cases, of course, it would be advantageous to consult the statistician. But as will appear from later discussion, there are certain types of problems of frequent occurrence which, while of a simple kind, possess such similarity of pattern that they could be discussed on a common basis. A few of such problems are discussed in this document in the hope that malaria workers may gain an insight not only into the type of reasoning the statistician employs in calculating the size or scope of any experiment but may also in simple cases be enabled to decide on the size of the sample himself.

The purpose of this section therefore is to set out the main statistical considerations as far as possible in a non-mathematical language with a view to offering assistance to malaria workers so that they can plan their experiments with proper regard to the minimum number of experimental subjects theoretically needed. Even though the statistical theory for the purpose involves the use of complicated mathematical formulae, so much simplification has already been made in its use that answers to many practical problems of frequent occurrence may be had without recourse to any calculation. For many cases ready-reckoning tables or graphical designs are available from which answers may be obtained merely at a glance. Simple graphical methods as well as some tables are described by means of which the size of the sample may be estimated without any calculations.

5.2   Objectives of Experimentation

Generally, the main objective of the experiment may belong to one of the two following categories:

1.   To compare the effects of two or more treatment procedures, as for instance when we wish to test whether the recovery rate among the treated malaria patients was significantly higher than among those not so treated.

2.   To obtain estimates of certain values with prescribed precision; for instance, to estimate the spleen rate of a community, (i.e. the percentage of children with enlarged spleen) with a $\pm$ 10% or $\pm$ error.

Most of the examples discussed in this document for both the above categories deal only with percentage values. Instead we may be interested in quantitative measures as, for instance, comparing increases in spleen size or measuring their average increase with desired precision from one period to another. Readers interested in the problem of determining sample sizes for quantitative measures are referred to Snedecor (1956) sections 2.15 and 4.7.

In the first case an experiment is planned in the hope that if a real difference of magnitude of practical interest does exist, the experiment should establish the difference in a conclusive manner, or to be more specific, the experiment should clearly indicate whether or not a difference in the recovery rates of a predetermined order of magnitude did exist.   If, owing to faulty planning, as for instance choosing an inadequate number of subjects, it was found that no conclusive result could be obtained, the experiment would have to be regarded almost as a failure.

In the second case, consideration regarding the adequacy of sample size implies that the estimate we obtain should not be associated with a margin of experimental error greater than that previously stipulated.   In other words, the sample should be large enough to provide the desired estimate with prescribed precision.

These needs arise from the fact that in biological experiments there can be many sources of experimental error as well as bias which should be anticipated at the planning stage and taken care of by means of proper experimental design and an adequate size of sample.   The required sample size for the comparison of two percentage values is discussed in the next section, while that for estimation of a percentage value is explained in section 5.4

5.3   Comparison of Two Percentages or Two Response Rates

In connexion with the planning of the experiments which fall in the first category mentioned above, the statistician begins, as already mentioned in section 2.9, by postulating a hypothesis somewhat unpleasant to the experimenter that one treatment does not differ from the other against which it is being compared.   In statistical terminology this is called the "null" hypothesis (section 2.9).   The objective of planning the experiment then is to supply sufficient evidence to contradict this hypothesis if it is untenable.   In fact it is only when the experiment has provided statistically adequate evidence to the effect that the hypothesis is untenable that one can legitimately proceed to argue that one treatment was different from the other.

As an alternative hypothesis we may postulate that the new treatment is better than the one with which it is compared by at least a predetermined amount, such as producing at least 10% better recovery rate or adding at least a fixed number of units to the measurements recorded under the controlled treatment.

5.3.1   Two kinds of error

It is well known that in biological experiments, owing to the effect of various controllable and uncontrollable factors, a certain amount of variability in results is to be expected even where an experiment is repeated under identical conditions.   For instance, if two presumably identical groups of experimental subjects are treated in an identical manner, i.e. given the same treatment, as far as possible under the same experimental conditions, the response rates (for instance, percentages of recoveries) will probably still not be exactly the same.   The amount of difference in the two response rates under these circumstances would depend, partly on how similar the two groups of experimental subjects were and partly on the number of subjects chosen.   Theoretically, if we chose an infinitely large number of possibly identical subjects, we could expect to obtain fairly identical response rates also, but an experiment with an infinitely large number of subjects from a practical point of view is rather an impossibility.

Recognizing therefore that some difference in the two response rates is to be attributable to chance factors, the statistician tries to guard against two kinds of error in his consideration of prescribing an adequate size of the sample.

Error of the "first kind" would arise if we were inadvertently to accept the two response rates as significantly different from each other when in actual fact the two are practically the same.   This is measured by the probability of erroneously judging one method better than the other when in fact the two methods are equally good (or bad).

Error of the "second kind" would arise if we were to consider the two treatments as the same when in actual fact they are different.   In other words, we measure the probability that we will fail to judge one treatment better (or worse) than the other when in fact it is better (or worse).

In calculating an adequate size of the sample we may postulate that the error of the first kind should not have a probability of more than 5% (or to be more stringent not more than 1%).   This implies that the two treatments, if really alike, will be falsely judged significantly different from each other in about 5% of cases only (or in 1% in the more stringent case).

For the same reason, we may try to keep the error of the second kind low at 10%, i.e. we so try to select the number of subjects that the possibility of the error of the second kind does not exceed 10%.

Our object thus is so to choose the sample size that both kinds of error can be kept under control. Of course, it is possible to make only one of these two kinds of errors in any experiment but generally we have no means of determining in advance which error of the two is likely to be made.

5.3.2 Adequate sample size for comparison of two percentages

The calculation of an adequate number of subjects to satisfy the above two requirements does require some rough knowledge in advance of what the two response rates are likely to be. In other words, the statistician can calculate the required sample size if the problem posed is something on the following lines:

If the response rate in one group which we may call the comparison group is p_c (about 40% for instance) and in the other or experimental group is p_e (approximately 60% for instance), how large must be the number of subjects experimented upon in each of the two groups so that the difference in experimental results can emerge into statistical significance? The terminology of "comparison" and "experimental" is used only conventionally. The discussion will, of course, relate to other comparisons, such as between two drugs, diets, vaccines or operational techniques. The group may contain patients, animals or cultures.

Of course, the question posed in this manner is of little or no practical significance for the reason that the exact values of the two percentages are generally not known. Generally, however, the choice of the value p_c can be made with a fair degree of reliability, based upon previous experience with some standard method. The value of p_e is then chosen sufficiently above the value of p_c (or sufficiently below its value) for the difference to be one that it is important to detect if present. For theoretical purposes, moderate variations in the assumed values of p_c and p_e are not important, especially if p_c and p_e are affected alike under the conditions of the experiment. Therefore, while the calculation of an adequate sample size will no doubt depend on some prior knowledge of the two response percentages, in most practical cases some indication or guess as to the magnitude of these percentages or the expected difference would be available, as for example when one drug has been used for the treatment of cases of a particular disease for a long time and the hospital records have shown a case mortality figure of 60% and a new drug is discovered, it being claimed that this drug reduces the case mortality by more than 30%. In cases such as this we have a basis for calculating the minimum number of patients on whom the two drugs should be tried experimentally in order to compare their effectiveness satisfactorily.

The formula of general application for the calculation of the size of sample to be used for each treatment involves rather complicated mathematical functions and is not given here. For practical purposes, by assuming that the error of the first kind should not exceed 0.05 (5% probability) and the error of the second kind should not exceed 0.1 (10% probability); the following nomogram provides, almost at a glance, the number of subjects which could be considered adequate for each treatment (Fig. 33).

In using this nomogram all that is necessary is to hold a flat ruler across the two percentages shown on the two vertical lines marked A and B. The smaller percentage could be measured along the line A. If both percentages exceed 50% we could work with the difference of each from 100%. A line drawn through any two percentages will cut the middle line, marked N, at the point which indicates by the marked scale the number of subjects to be selected in each group. For example, if by the use of the standard treatment (comparison group) 30% recovery rate has been experienced in the past and we wish to compare it with another treatment which is expected to raise the recovery rate to 60% or more, we draw a line through points marked 30% and 60% on the A and B scales. The line marked N is thus cut at the point marked 50 which indicates that we need a minimum of 50 experimental subjects in each of the two groups.

If a more precise estimate of sample size is needed, or if we need estimates for risks other than 5% and 10% (probabilities of errors of the first and second kind), reference should be made to W. A. Wallis (see Eisenhart et al., 1947).

5.4   Estimating Percentages with Prescribed Precision

The problem discussed in this section is best illustrated by a typical example, namely that of determining the spleen rate of children in a community by choosing a sufficiently large number of children for the rate to be estimated with less than say $\pm$ 10% error.   A similar problem would arise also if we were to estimate the recovery rate of a homogeneous group of patients with a disease, all of whom had had the same treatment administered to them.   In sample surveys it may be desirable to estimate the prevalence rate (percentage of persons found suffering from the disease at any time), the problem being to ascertain how many individuals should be examined for the estimated percentage not to be grossly in error.   The need for obtaining such estimates of percentages is indeed very general and many more instances would suggest themselves to the reader, depending on the field of study. The sample size may of course depend upon the facilities available and the amount of precision required for the estimate.   It is well known that the estimate obtained from a sample is more likely to be near the truth if we examine a large sample than if we examine only a small one.   The important question always arises, how many units should we examine in order to be reasonably sure that our result will not differ from the unknown truth by a given percentage error?   In other words, what should be the sample size to ensure that the percentage we estimate is a "reasonable precise estimate of the true percentage"?

The term "reasonably precise" used here needs clarification.   In the first place, we should specify in advance the maximum allowable range of error in the estimate or the precision with which we wish to estimate.   For instance, if we are interested in estimating the spleen rate among children, we may specify in advance that the estimated rate should not differ from the true spleen rate (the one that we would obtain if all the children in the population could be examined) by more than say $\pm$ 10% or $\pm$ 5% or $\pm$ 1%, etc.

Secondly, we must recognize that absolute certainty that this range of error will never be exceeded is a theoretical impossibility.   All the same, by choosing a sufficiently large sample we can be reasonably sure that the prescribed range of error will not be exceeded.   For this purpose, what we usually do is to stipulate

FIG. 33   NOMOGRAM FOR ESTIMATING THE SAMPLE SIZE FOR COMPARING TWO PERCENTAGES

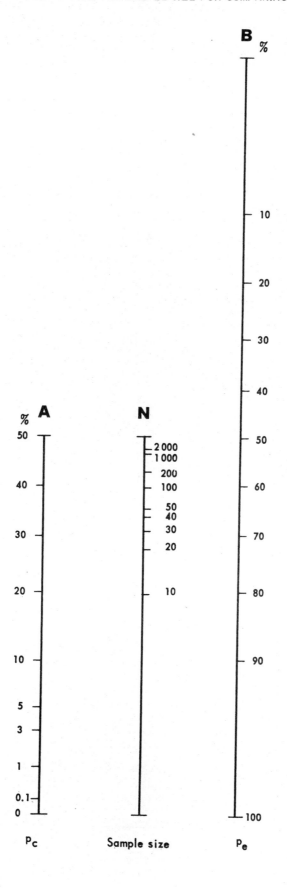

in advance that the prescribed error will not be exceeded by say a probability of five in a 100 (or to be more exacting, by a probability of one in a 100). In other words, we stipulate that the probability is 95% (or 99%) that the estimate we obtain from the sample will not differ from the true value by more than the range of error prescribed. Of course we may set any limit of probability but the convention is to demand that in not more than five cases out of 100 (or one in a 100) shall our estimate differ from the true value by the stipulated error. In statistical language therefore, the term "reasonable precision" may mean that the probability of being in error from the true population figure by more than a stipulated percentage is as small as 5% (or 1%). The term therefore contains an idea of degree.

The determination of the adequacy of sample size therefore involves the following four considerations:

1. <u>The precision with which we wish to obtain the estimate.</u> The narrower the range of error prescribed the larger should our sample be. To some extent of course the specification of error will depend upon the extent of the accuracy needed and the limitation of results.

2. <u>The degree of sureness with which we wish to obtain the precision.</u> For 99% certainty we need a larger sample than for 95% certainty.

3. <u>The roughly estimated value of the percentage in the whole population or region under consideration.</u>

4. <u>The manner in which the sample is chosen from the total population.</u> It is only by drawing a random sample that we can determine the sampling error.

In regard to the third consideration above, it is helpful if, either on a <u>priori</u> grounds or based on past experience, we have some idea in advance, even if only approximate, of the magnitude of the percentage we actually want to estimate. In cases which generally arise in practice we do possess some inkling of what the percentage is expected to be. Such a figure, not unusually based on guesswork, is of course the only information we can use in estimating the sample size.

The fourth consideration above emphasizes the fact that the sample drawn should be strictly random.   If any other scheme of sampling is adopted the size of the sample to be chosen will be different, and we have to make sure that there is no conscious or unconscious bias which is likely to vitiate the results.   In statistical language, the word "random" connotes a specific method which has already been explained in section 2.20.1.   At the risk of repetition it may be emphasized that even an adequately chosen sample will not be able to compensate for inaccuracies in experiment such as those arising from faulty observation or wrong classification of the subject.

Statistical theory also distinguishes between selected sample sizes which are comparatively small in relation to the total number of things in existence compared with relatively large samples.   In many cases, the total number of things is so large that for theoretical purposes we can presume it to be infinite, as for instance the blood in a patient's body in relation to the blood sample taken to study a patient's leucocytes.   Again, in the study of the sex ratio at birth in countries, the number of children born may be presumed infinitely large in relation to the size of sample generally needed for this estimate.   But cases do occur where the total number of things cannot be presumed to be infinitely large.   For instance, we may wish to estimate by sampling process the percentage of children with an enlarged spleen in a village which may have only 100 children.   Obviously by selecting 50 children out of a total of 100 one would approach much nearer the spleen rate for that village than if that village had 1000 children and again only 50 were examined.   We therefore discuss separately the problem of sampling from "finite" population as compared with sampling from "infinite" population.

It should be noted that in so far as the computation of adequate sample size is based on some previous estimation of the population percentage, the sample size thus obtained may fail to provide the desired degree of precision owing to imprecise estimation of the population percentage made before commencement of the experiment. Or, on the other hand, the computed sample size may happen to be greater than what would have been adequate.   Thus, although the discussions in the following sections should provide satisfactory methods of determining the adequate sample size, these methods should not be regarded as providing the desired size exactly.

5.4.1   Sampling from an infinite population or proportionately small samples

Ready-reckoning tables prepared by Ross & Stott (1911) for sampling from an infinite population were based on statistical theory judged appropriate at that time. In recent years certain weaknesses of the theory have been taken care of, thus rendering it unnecessary to have to make certain approximations which facilitated the work of Ross and Stott.   These authors had assumed that the error around the true value was expected to be of the same magnitude on either side, i.e. the so-called ± errors were presumed by them to be of similar or equal probability of occurrence. That this is not usually the case when dealing with small samples will be obvious from the following simple example.   Let us suppose that the actual value of spleen rate in a large population is 10%.   If the size of the random sample chosen is very small (say 10 children only), then on the average we would expect one child out of every 10 to show enlargement of spleen.   Owing to errors of sampling, however, the sample estimate may err on both sides of this true value.   Thus, if no child shows enlarged spleen in the sample we would get an observed rate of 0% (a 10% error on the minus side), but we cannot possibly make a larger error in this direction. On the positive side however, the possible range of error is from 20% upwards, depending upon whether we find 2, 3, 4, ... children with enlarged spleen in our sample.   From the theory of probability we also find that the chance of observing percentage values of 20, 30 and over is also quite high.   Thus, while on the negative side we can at most have an error of minus 10%, on the positive side errors of higher magnitudes are also to be expected.   As a matter of fact, it is only when the actual percentage in the population is around 50 that we can expect the errors from sampling to be of about equal magnitude with both positive and negative signs.   Theoretically, similar equality is expected when the size of the sample is very large, but it will be clear that in the case of rather samll samples generally met with in practice, we should think of the possibility of unequal magnitudes of error around the true value.   Bearing this consideration in mind, we present a series of charts (Figs. 34 to 39) and ready-reckoning tables (Tables 48 and 49) to facilitate the selection of a sample size so that the range of error can be limited within a permissible extent.   The use of these charts and tables is explained below.

Table 48 shows the values of the upper and lower limits (called the confidence limits) between which the true percentage value of the population is likely to fall in 95% cases. The table covers cases when different sized samples are drawn and sets out the confidence limits corresponding to various percentage values observed in the sample. For instance, if we examined a sample of 80 children and found 30% children with enlarged spleen, Table 48 tells us that the true population percentage is likely to lie somewhere between 20% and 41%. Thus this table may be used to judge the range of population value (confidence interval) after the experiment or survey has been carried out, i.e. once the sample percentage is known. This table may also be used for the purpose of determining an adequate sample size for each particular survey. For this purpose we first make a rough guess on the population percentage value in question on the basis of past experience or some relevant information. If, for example, we are concerned with estimating spleen rate in a child population and if the rate is roughly guessed at about 30%, we look at the column headed 30% and find the various confidence limits corresponding to different tentative sample sizes. Thus for instance corresponding to the hypothetically observed value of 30% and the sample size of 80 we find in Table 48, that the confidence interval is from 20% to 41%. If this is considered too large a range then we look at the figures corresponding to sample size of say 200. The range is then reduced to 24% - 38%. Thus stipulating in advance what our permissible range of error is to be, we can with the help of this table read the required sample size.

Table 49 is similar to Table 48, but corresponds to 99% certainty. It is seen that, for the same sample size and observed percentage, the confidence interval is wider for Table 49 than for Table 48.

Table 48. Confidence intervals at 95% probability level corresponding to varying sample sizes and sample percentages

Sample size	Percentage observed in sample										
	5%	10%	20%	30%	40%	50%	60%	70%	80%	90%	95%
10	*	0 - 45	3 - 56	7 - 65	12 - 74	19 - 81	26 - 88	35 - 93	44 - 98	56 - 100	*
20	0 - 25	1 - 32	6 - 44	12 - 54	19 - 64	27 - 73	36 - 81	46 - 88	56 - 94	68 - 99	75 - 100
30	*	2 - 26	8 - 39	15 - 49	23 - 59	31 - 69	41 - 77	51 - 85	61 - 92	74 - 98	*
40	1 - 17	3 - 24	9 - 35	17 - 47	25 - 57	34 - 66	43 - 75	53 - 83	65 - 91	76 - 97	83 - 99
50	*	3 - 22	10 - 34	18 - 45	26 - 55	36 - 65	45 - 74	55 - 82	66 - 90	78 - 97	*
60	1 - 14	3 - 20	11 - 32	19 - 43	28 - 54	37 - 63	46 - 72	57 - 81	68 - 89	80 - 97	86 - 99
80	1 - 12	4 - 19	12 - 30	20 - 41	29 - 51	39 - 61	49 - 71	59 - 80	70 - 88	81 - 96	88 - 99
100	2 - 11	5 - 18	13 - 29	21 - 40	30 - 50	40 - 60	50 - 70	60 - 79	71 - 87	82 - 95	89 - 98
200	2 - 9	6 - 14	16 - 26	24 - 38	33 - 47	43 - 57	53 - 67	62 - 76	74 - 84	86 - 94	91 - 98
300	3 - 8	7 - 14	16 - 25	25 - 36	35 - 46	44 - 56	54 - 65	64 - 75	75 - 84	86 - 93	92 - 97
400	3 - 8	7 - 13	16 - 24	26 - 35	35 - 45	45 - 55	55 - 65	65 - 74	76 - 84	87 - 93	92 - 97
500	3 - 7	8 - 13	17 - 24	26 - 34	36 - 44	46 - 54	56 - 64	66 - 74	76 - 83	87 - 92	93 - 97
1000	4 - 7	8 - 12	18 - 23	27 - 33	37 - 43	47 - 53	57 - 63	67 - 73	77 - 82	88 - 92	93 - 96

* unexpected case

Table 49.   Confidence intervals at 99% probability level corresponding to varying sample sizes and sample percentages

Sample size	Percentage observed in sample										
	5%	10%	20%	30%	40%	50%	60%	70%	80%	90%	95%
10	*	0 - 54	1 - 65	4 - 74	8 - 81	13 - 87	19 - 92	26 - 96	35 - 99	46 -100	*
20	0 - 32	1 - 39	4 - 51	8 - 61	15 - 70	22 - 78	30 - 85	39 - 92	49 - 96	61 - 99	68 -100
30	*	1 - 32	5 - 44	11 - 55	18 - 65	26 - 74	35 - 82	45 - 89	56 - 95	68 - 99	*
40	0 - 21	2 - 28	7 - 41	13 - 51	21 - 61	30 - 70	39 - 79	49 - 87	59 - 93	72 - 98	79 -100
50	*	2 - 26	8 - 38	15 - 49	23 - 59	32 - 68	41 - 77	51 - 85	62 - 92	74 - 98	*
60	1 - 17	3 - 24	9 - 36	16 - 47	24 - 57	33 - 67	43 - 76	53 - 84	64 - 91	76 - 97	83 - 99
80	1 - 15	3 - 22	10 - 34	18 - 45	26 - 55	36 - 64	45 - 74	55 - 82	66 - 90	78 - 97	85 - 99
100	1 - 14	4 - 20	11 - 32	19 - 43	28 - 53	37 - 63	47 - 72	57 - 81	68 - 89	80 - 96	86 - 99
200	2 - 11	5 - 17	13 - 28	22 - 39	31 - 49	41 - 59	51 - 69	61 - 78	72 - 87	83 - 95	89 - 98
300	2 - 9	6 - 15	14 - 27	23 - 37	33 - 47	43 - 57	53 - 67	63 - 77	73 - 86	85 - 94	91 - 98
400	3 - 9	7 - 14	15 - 26	24 - 36	34 - 46	44 - 56	54 - 66	64 - 76	74 - 85	85 - 94	91 - 98
500	3 - 8	7 - 14	16 - 25	25 - 36	34 - 46	44 - 56	54 - 66	64 - 75	75 - 84	86 - 93	92 - 97
1000	3 - 7	8 - 13	17 - 24	26 - 34	36 - 44	46 - 54	56 - 64	66 - 74	76 - 83	87 - 92	93 - 97

* unexpected case

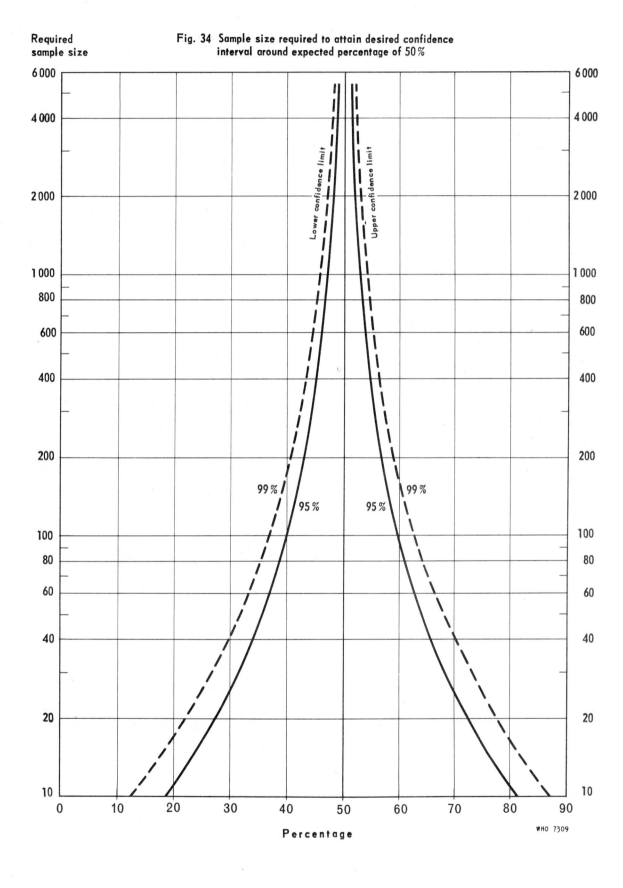

Required sample size

Fig. 34 Sample size required to attain desired confidence interval around expected percentage of 50 %

Lower confidence limit

Upper confidence limit

99 % 95 %   95 % 99 %

Percentage

WHO 7309

Required
sample size

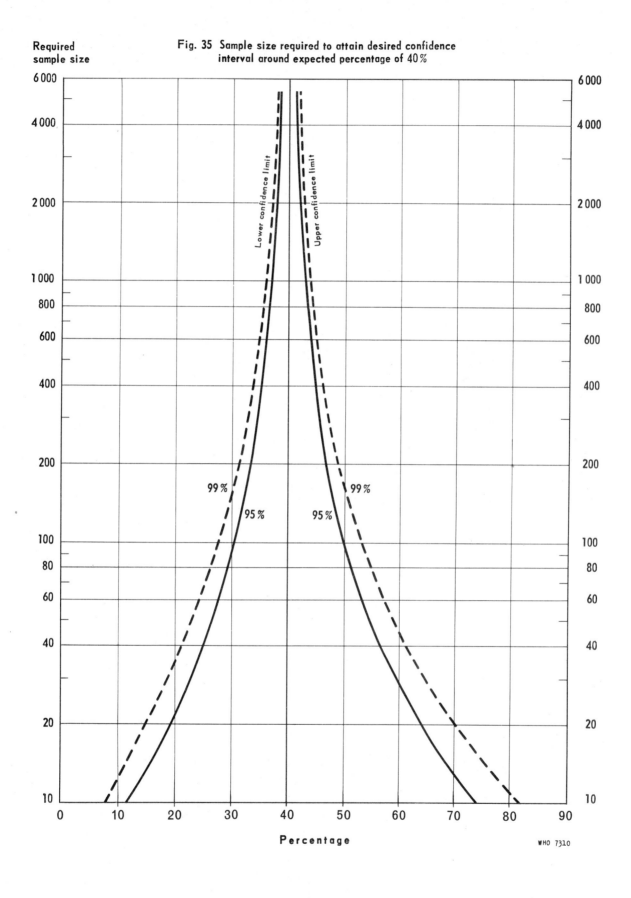

Fig. 35 Sample size required to attain desired confidence
interval around expected percentage of 40 %

Lower confidence limit

Upper confidence limit

99 %

95 %

95 %

99 %

Percentage

WHO 7310

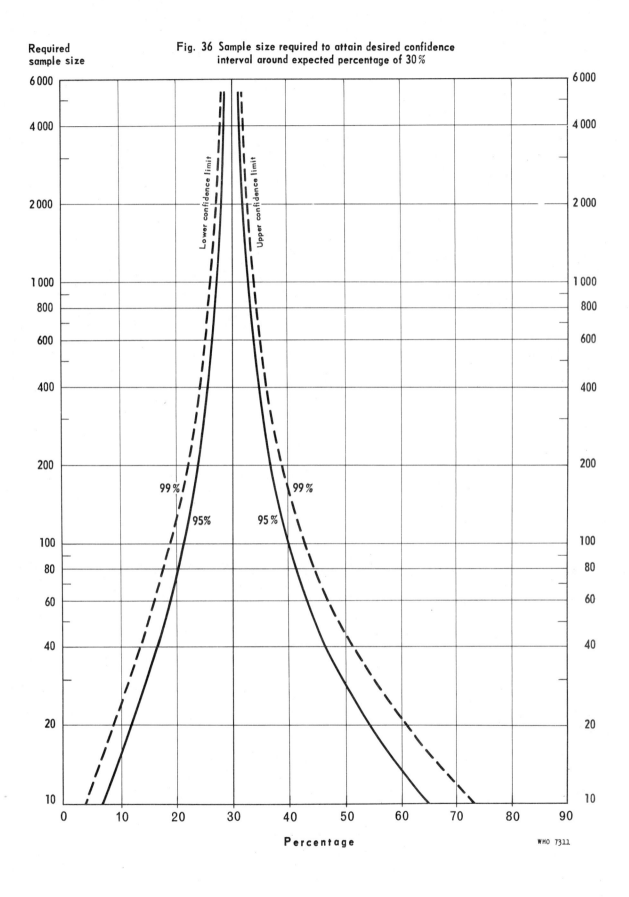

Required sample size

Fig. 36 Sample size required to attain desired confidence interval around expected percentage of 30%

Lower confidence limit

Upper confidence limit

99%   99%

95%   95%

Percentage

WHO 7311

Required sample size

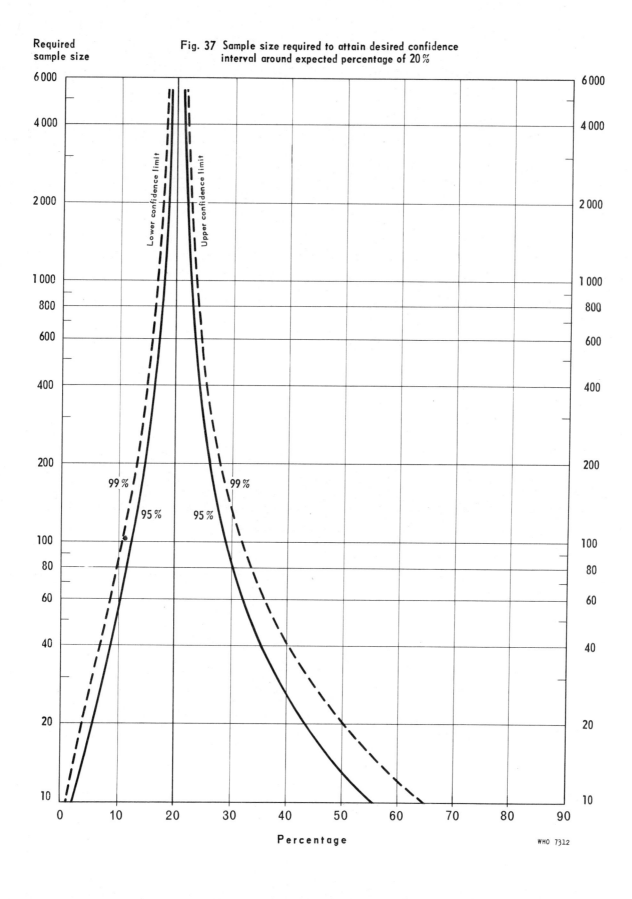

Lower confidence limit

Upper confidence limit

99 %

99 %

95 %

95 %

Percentage

WHO 7312

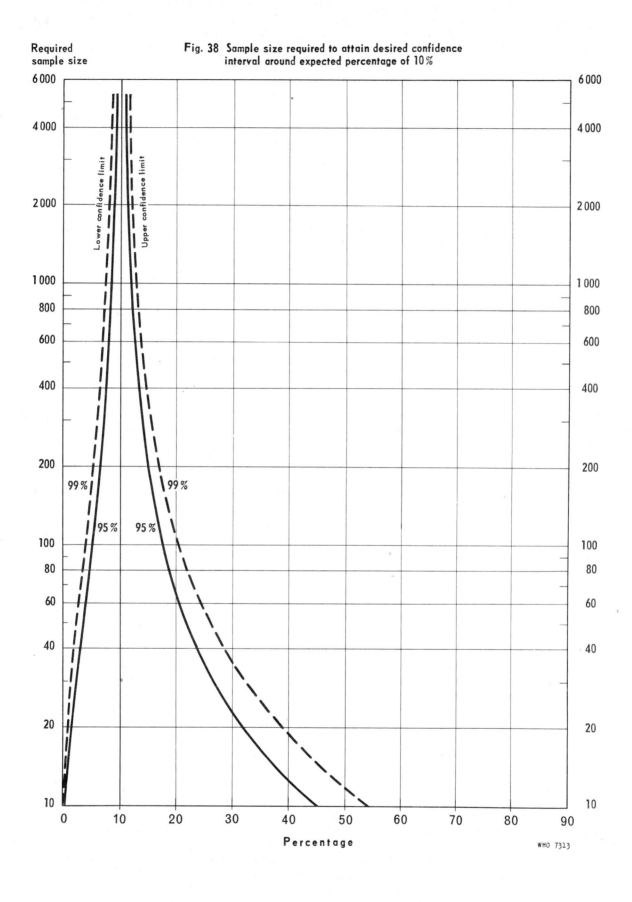

Fig. 38 Sample size required to attain desired confidence interval around expected percentage of 10 %

Required sample size

Percentage

Lower confidence limit

Upper confidence limit

WHO 7313

**Required
sample size**

Fig. 39 Sample size required to attain desired confidence
interval around expected percentage of 5%

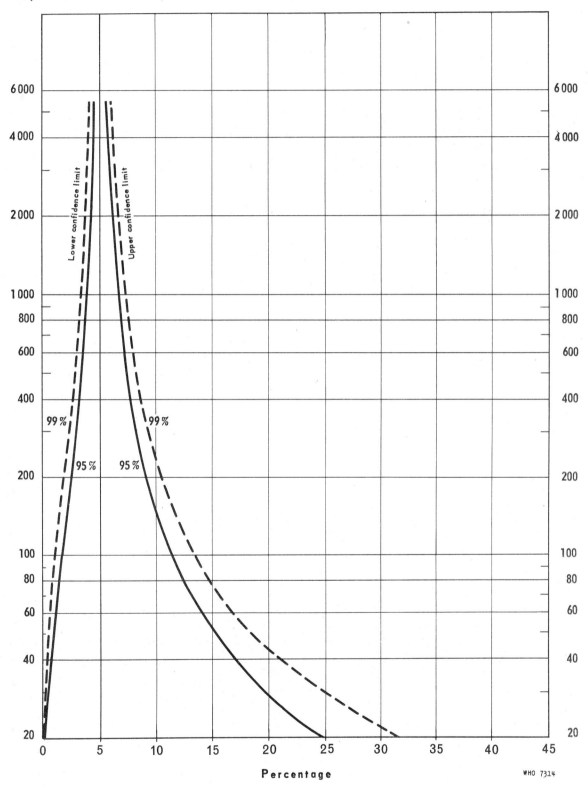

Percentage

WHO 7314

A series of charts are also given to facilitate the same estimation of the size of sample.   Fig. 34 for instance relates to the case where in the actual population we expect a spleen rate - or for that matter any other percentage - to be of the order of about 50%.   Along the horizontal scale are shown the percentages, and the vertical scale shows the corresponding sample size.   The two curved lines running on either side of the 50% vertical line mark the two lower and upper confidence limits of error from the sample.   The continuous lines relate to 95% probability level and the dotted lines to 99% probability.   As the sample size decreases these curves have a tendency to widen out.   On the other hand, the interval is narrowed by choosing larger and larger samples.   Theoretically of course, both these curves will meet the 50% point if the sample was infinitely large, that is, if we examine the whole population.   As an example of its use, if at the 95% probability level we want about 10% error on either side, then we can see that the curved lines cross the 40% and 60% values when the sample size is 100.   A 20% error on either side is expected when the sample size is 26 individuals.   This chart relates to the case where the percentage or the rate expected in the sample is of the order of 50%. The charts which follow (Figs. 35 to 39) cover cases where the rates are of the order of 40%, 30%, 20%, 10% and 5% respectively and can be used in the same manner as in the example given above for the 50% chart.   If the expected percentage is in excess of 50% we could take the difference from 100 and look up the corresponding chart.

5.4.2   Sampling from a finite population or proportionately large samples

As stated in section 5.4, if the entire population or things under consideration are relatively limited we will obtain greater precision in our estimate than if the same sized sample were drawn from an infinitely large population.   In other words, to attain required precision the sample size (obtained by using the formula for an infinite population) should be reduced when dealing with a finite population.   This can be approximately achieved by multiplying the sample size required for an infinite population (given already in Tables 48 and 49) by a correction factor whose value will be less than one.   In Table 50 the value of this correction factor is given corresponding to varying values of the percentage which the sample size required for an infinite population bears to the total finite population. For instance, if it is found from Table 48 that for the required precision a sample size for an infinite population should be 300 and our finite population is only 200 then the percentage of this sample size to available population is (300/200) x 100% or 150%. The correction factor corresponding to 150% as read from Table 50 is 0.40 which multiplied by 300 gives the value 120 for the sample size required.

As another example let us say that in a community the total number of children available is 250 and we want the spleen rate to be estimated with about $\pm$ 10% error. Reference to Table 48 given in Section 5.4.1 shows that assuming the spleen rate to be of the order of 40% we would require about 100 children if we were sampling from an infinitely large number of children. In the present case the sample size 100 constitutes 40% of the available number of children, namely 250. The following table shows that the correction factor corresponding to 40% is 0.71. Therefore our sample size should be 100 multiplied by 0.71, that is, we should examine 71 children out of 250 to obtain a precision of $\pm$ 10% around the expected spleen rate.

Table 50. Correction factor for sampling from a finite population

Percentage of the sample size for infinite population to the finite population size	Correction factor by which to multiply the sample size for infinite population to obtain sample size for finite population
0	1.00
5	.95
10	.91
15	.87
20	.83
25	.80
30	.77
35	.74
40	.71
45	.69
50	.67
55	.65
60	.63
65	.61
70	.59
75	.57
80	.56
85	.54
90	.53
95	.51

Table 50 (Continued)

Percentage of the sample size for infinite population to the finite population size	Correction factor by which to multiply the sample size for infinite population to obtain sample size for finite population
100	.50
105	.49
110	.48
115	.47
120	.45
125	.44
130	.43
135	.43
140	.42
145	.41
150	.40
160	.38
170	.37
180	.36
190	.34
200	.33
210	.32
220	.31
230	.30
240	.29
250	.29
260	.28
270	.27
280	.26
290	.26
300	.25
310	.24
320	.24
330	.23
340	.23
350	.22
360	.22
370	.21
380	.21
390	.20
400	.20
425	.19
450	.18
475	.17
500	.17

Although this table has been extended to cover the range from 0% to 500% it will readily be apparent that when the sample size required for an infinite population is very large as compared with the finite population available, as would be the case when we are seeking a high degree of precision, then we may have to sample something like 70% to 90% of the finite population. The real purpose of sampling of course is to keep the number relatively low as compared to the population available. Therefore in case the demands of high precision necessitate a sampling of say more than 70% of the entire population, it may seem advantageous to examine the entire population rather than a sample of it.

5.5 Size of Sample Required for Inspection of Products (Control of Consumer's Risk)

As an example of the type of problems discussed in this section, let us suppose that a lot of DDT spray-pumps are offered for inspection. Those that are defective will blow up at a certain pressure. It would be impracticable to examine each item to ensure that they pass a prescribed hydrostatic test. The problem then is to find the minimum number to be tested as a sample in order to have at least 95% certainty that in the whole lot the defective items do not constitute more than say 1% or 5% or 10%.

The number of items to be included in a randomly drawn sample will depend, of course, on how large the entire lot is as well as on the prescribed minimum number of defectives which we are willing to accept. For instance, the larger the size of the entire lot the larger should our sample be. However, it is a mistaken belief that the sample size should be exactly proportional to the size of the lot. As will be clear from Table 51 the sample size is not related in direct proportion to the lot size. Again we need a relatively smaller sample if we are prepared to accept up to 10% defective pumps than if our maximum acceptable limit of defectives is fixed as low as 1%. The sample size will also depend upon how certain we wish to be in our test. If we want to have 99% certainty that the prescribed acceptable limit of defectives is not exceeded, then we need a relatively larger sample than if we wanted to be only 95% sure of rejecting a defective lot.

Table 51 shows the sample size adequate for carrying out tests corresponding to varying size of the lot as well as to the maximum percentage of defectives to be accepted by the test. The table gives sample sizes separately for 95%, 90%, 80% and 70% certainty of rejecting the lot if it contains more than the prescribed percentage of defectives. It must be noted that we are here considering only the risk to the user, i.e. we are ensuring that the user of the items is not supplied with a lot of less than a specified quality. The tables should not be used in the event of our being interested in the producer's risk, that is, the risk of erroneously rejecting by sample test the lot that does in fact meet with the prescribed specification. If our interest lies also in reducing the producer's risk the sample size will have to be relatively larger. The rule to be adopted is that if the sample of the size indicated in the table shows even a single defective item the entire lot is to be rejected. On the other hand, if no defective item is found in the sample, the whole lot is to be regarded as of acceptable quality. It is emphasized that the sample drawn should be strictly at random.

Table 51

Table showing the size of the sample to be tested to ensure 95%, 90%,
80% and 70% certainty of not accepting an unsatisfactory lot
(The entire lot is to be rejected if even a single unit in the sample
is found defective)

95% certainty

Size of the Lot	Maximum percentage of defectives to be permitted in the lot					
	1%	5%	10%	20%	30%	40%
100	95	45	25	13	9	6
500	225	56	28	14	9	6
1000	258	57	29	14	9	6
5000	290	59	29	14	9	6
Infinite	299	59	29	14	9	6

90% certainty

Size of the Lot	Maximum percentage of defectives to be permitted in the lot					
	1%	5%	10%	20%	30%	40%
100	90	37	20	10	7	5
500	184	43	22	11	7	5
1000	205	44	22	11	7	5
5000	224	45	22	11	7	5
Infinite	230	45	22	11	7	5

80% certainty

Size of the Lot	Maximum percentage of defectives to be permitted in the lot					
	1%	5%	10%	20%	30%	40%
100	80	27	15	7	5	4
500	138	31	16	8	5	4
1000	148	31	16	8	5	4
5000	158	32	16	8	5	4
Infinite	161	32	16	8	5	4

70% certainty

Size of the Lot	Maximum percentage of defectives to be permitted in the lot					
	1%	5%	10%	20%	30%	40%
100	70	21	11	6	4	3
500	107	23	12	6	4	3
1000	113	24	12	6	4	3
5000	119	24	12	6	4	3
Infinite	120	24	12	6	4	3

6.   REFERENCE IN THE TEXT TO CURRENT PROBLEMS AND THEIR STATISTICAL APPROACH

An attempt is made in this section to indicate appropriate section references to discussion of the statistical considerations involved and the suggested methodology applicable in some of the problems frequently encountered by malaria workers.

6.1 Malariometric Rates

1.   Comparison of malariometric rates from two villages:

χ^2 test: Section 2.11

2.   Comparison of spleen size before and after spraying operations:

Contingency tables, Section 2.11

3.   Number of subjects to be examined to obtain desired degree of precision in the rate: Section 5.4

4.   Method of selecting a sample of children for examination: Section 2.20.1

5.   Endemicity of malaria: Section 4.7.3

6.2 Vital and Health Statistics Data

1.   Rates, ratios and indices used: Section 3.3

2.   Time series: Section 2.22

3.   Standardization of data: Section 3.6

6.3 Chemotherapeutic Experiments

1.   Methods of planning chemotherapeutic experiments:

Section 5.1 and 5.2

2.   Number of individuals to be included in the trial when comparing two treatments:

Section 5.3.2

3.   Sampling: Section 2.20

6.4   Malaria Demonstration Projects

    1.   Statistical information to be collected: Section 4.4

    2.   Planning of malaria control projects: Section 4.3

6.5   Malaria Eradication: Section 4.7

6.6   Resistance to Insecticides

    1.   Estimation of LD_{50} or LC_{50}: Section 2.21

6.7   Preparation of Statistical Reports

    1.   Collection of data: Section 2.1; Section 2.2; Section 2.3

    2.   Presentation of data by tables: Section 2.4

    3.   Charts and diagrams: Section 2.6

    4.   Interpretation and analysis: Section 4.5

6.8   Appraisal and evaluation: Section 4.6

    1.   Collection and classification of data: Sections 2.1, 2.2 and 2.3.

APPENDIX A

LOGARITHMS

An elementary understanding of the use of logarithms is necessary for the analysis of data collected in connexion with malaria studies or surveys. After giving a brief explanation of the underlying theory, a number of instances are given below when logarithms will be found useful in connexion with problems arising in malaria work.

Let us suppose that $10^x = X$ and $10^y = Y$. For instance, if $x = 2$ and $y = 3$, $10^x = 100$ and $10^y = 1000$. The indices x and y are called the logarithms of the numbers X and Y. Logarithms therefore are the powers of 10 (or of any other base if so desired) corresponding to the larger quantities X and Y.

Since $10^x \times 10^y$ is equal to 10^{x+y} we may note that if we want to multiply the two quantities X and Y, we can do so also by simply adding the corresponding x and y, and finding out what the number given by 10^{x+y} corresponds to. The numbers corresponding to 10^x, 10^y or 10^{x+y} can easily be looked up in published tables of logarithms (J. Pryde, ed. 1948).

The two advantages of this procedure are that:

(i) addition of two numbers is always easier to perform than multiplication, and

(ii) the numbers x and y are always relatively much smaller in magnitude than X and Y, and therefore sometimes easier to handle. There are, in fact, many other advantages of working with small x and y which may correspond to larger X and Y.

Since 10^3 is 1000
10^2 is 100
10^1 is 10
10^0 is 1

we may note that the logarithm of 1000 is 3
"   "   " 100 is 2
"   "   " 10 is 1
"   "   " 1 is 0

Appendix A

It is also clear from the above that for numbers lying between 1 and 10 the logarithms will be a fractional quantity. For numbers lying between 10 and 100 the value of the logarithm will be between 1 and 2, i.e. digit 1 followed by a decimal part. For numbers lying between 100 and 1000 the logarithm will lie between 2 and 3, i.e. it will begin with digit 2 followed by a decimal part.

The decimal part of a logarithm is called the mantissa, and the integral part is called the characteristic. It will be observed that the characteristic will always be one less than the number of digits in the original number. Thus, the characteristic for the number 97 will be 1, because this number has two digits. The characteristic for 975 will be 2, etc. The characteristic for 9.75 will be 0, because the number has only one digit before the decimal part. For fractional quantities the characteristic is expressed as a negative integer, and as a rule mantissa is always expressed as a positive fraction. As a general rule, the characteristic for decimal fractions is a negative quantity and is one more than the number of zeros following the decimal point. The following table giving negative values of characteristic and positive values of mantissa illustrates this. Inasmuch as only the characteristic is a negative quantity and not the mantissa, the negative sign is placed above the characteristic and not preceding it.

Number	Logarithm
1	0.000
.5	$\bar{1}$.69897
.05	$\bar{2}$.69897
.005	$\bar{3}$.69897
.0005	$\bar{4}$.69897

So long as the digits in the number do not change the mantissa remains the same. Thus, for example, the quantities 316 or 31.6 or 0.0316 will all have the same mantissa, but the characteristics will be 2, 1, or $\bar{2}$ respectively.

Number	Logarithm
316	2.49969
31.6	1.49969
0.0316	$\bar{2}$.49969

Since the mantissa remains the same, it is only the value of the mantissa that have been tabulated in most of the tables of logarithms, it being expected that the characteristic will be added by inspection of the figures. For example, if we require logarithm of 0.097 we find from the published table that the mantissa corresponding to digits 97 is 98677. The logarithm of the quantities 0.097 therefore, is given by $\bar{2}$.98677.

Use of logarithms

The facility that logarithms offer for carrying out multiplication has already been mentioned. We may illustrate this by numerical example. To multiply 45 by 0.36 we have merely to add the logarithm of 45 and 0.36, i.e. we add the two quantities 1.65321 and $\bar{1}$.55630, as read out from the table of logarithms and get:

$$1.65321 + \bar{1}.55630 = 1.65321 + (-1 + .55630)$$
$$= 1.65321 - 1 + .55630$$
$$= 1.20951$$

Since the characteristic here is 1, it means that the product will consist of two digits. The number corresponding to the mantissa 20951 is 1620. We place a decimal after two digits and the value of the product is 16.20.

The use of logarithms in carrying out divisions may be illustrated on the same figures. For instance, if we want to divide 16.2 by 0.36, all we have to do is to subtract the logarithm of 0.36 from the logarithm of 16.2 i.e. subtract the quantity $\bar{1}$.55630 from 1.20951 and get:

Appendix A

$$1.20951 - \bar{1}.55630 = 1.20951 - (-1 + .55630)$$
$$= 1.20951 + 1 - .55630$$
$$= 1.65321$$

The number corresponding to this logarithm, i.e. its anti-logarithm, will have two digits, because the characteristic is 1. The mantissa 65321 corresponds therefore to the number 45.

Logarithms are useful for finding out powers of quantities such as squares, cubes, fourth power, etc. They are almost indispensable for finding out roots, square roots, cube roots, or higher roots. To find out the power of any quantity (integral or fractional) the rule is to multiply the logarithm of the original number by the power, and find the corresponding anti-log. For instance, to find the sixth root of the quantity 729 we divide the logarithm of 729, i.e. 2.86273 by 6, and get 0.47712. The characteristic being 0, the figure will be only one digit. The mantissa 47712 corresponds to the digit 3, which therefore is the sixth root of the quantity 729.

In connexion with the calculation of the geometric mean in section 2.11 it was stated that we have to find the nth root of the products of all the measurements. Thus, to find the geometric mean of the 15 measurements given in section 2.11, we proceed by adding their logarithms (a step that is necessary in connexion with the finding of the products), and divide by 15 to find the 15th root as follows:

Measurement	Logarithms
1.80	0.25527
1.74	0.24055
1.85	0.26717
1.53	0.18469
1.89	0.27646
1.96	0.29226
1.82	0.26007

Measurement (Contd.)	Logarithms (Contd.)
1.82	0.26007
1.97	0.29447
1.97	0.29447
2.00	0.30103
1.95	0.29003
1.97	0.29885
1.93	0.28556
2.10	0.32222
Total	4.12317

The total of the 15 logarithms is 4.12317.

To find the geometric mean we divide this total logarithm by 15 (the number of measurements) and get 0.27488. The corresponding logarithm is 1.88, which is therefore the geometric mean of the observations.

Another important use of the logarithms is in connexion with the charting of curves showing incidence of disease as already described in section 2.5.

An important point to note in this connexion is that by using logarithmic scale we do not measure absolute changes but only relative changes from one period to another. A constant difference along the logarithmic scale means a steady proportionate change which is entirely independent of the magnitude of the quantity measured. This fact is of considerably use in malaria work. For instance, if mosquito traps are placed in the same area they may differ markedly in the gross levels of catches. A trap near a breeding place may yield several times the number of mosquitos which may happen to be caught in traps less favourably placed. The same argument would, of course, apply to catches of adult mosquitos made by any other method. A record of the catches at periodic intervals will therefore show considerable variation. But if catches for the two or more traps are charted on the same logarithmic scale, we could at a glance study relative changes. In other

words, the question of the efficiency of traps will not enter into any comparisons
made with respect to time.

For the same reason, it would be found convenient to chart malaria cases and
deaths on a log-scale, to study whether the two vary in constant proportion in time
or not.   The same scale is also found useful for studying relative changes in
malaria cases versus PUO (pyrexia of uncertain origin).

APPENDIX B

RANDOM SAMPLING NUMBERS

10374	81242	54237	47830	14309	03811	02339	15824
62345	80164	13387	63042	04736	81875	09086	84918
57668	07422	79716	92342	39648	54201	12307	20120
67015	68827	98912	83977	29847	93797	34722	28708
36283	79784	33025	81697	33254	33383	50361	75978
55866	32817	36969	38994	42853	32317	92865	33540
69534	38515	74323	62723	42768	45728	25454	24516
97409	87760	27354	52549	61977	17976	87474	77875
00905	91777	94373	48733	79688	05266	30331	96540
10731	38217	00252	84837	86644	60575	08220	30842
83219	96115	87128	88134	56039	04789	77119	45069
85563	08858	91872	82309	44923	53422	54141	46367
04928	68671	70215	16585	87309	60063	24182	56908
43105	80571	31869	56940	34376	31135	83453	19234
52262	35954	60506	34199	05865	81436	62723	73125
44163	39334	24705	34712	70991	83012	31553	22885
01762	36247	15408	20976	44133	76487	67438	36070
10622	72751	92283	51674	58183	82486	27401	50038
21687	48047	68835	61150	68582	86993	71551	64538
72005	96260	96382	98559	34991	42317	96840	46302
48977	51839	25511	19005	28907	68216	48859	87504
06636	42542	01208	26486	34318	22036	17945	07995
48393	80704	25749	32934	30569	18154	71595	01489
11011	07502	63076	70490	63323	85238	03724	70326
00441	29608	10669	83143	12853	33939	43893	34830
22539	33440	05274	58865	04486	05836	10857	42014
69428	79218	69384	08697	50724	27186	66327	54830
76833	41926	41642	30052	22811	48325	63545	56267
93092	96685	15674	28554	75784	93604	40430	71889
15306	29811	21251	31591	94832	25038	32750	65690
20173	91869	12150	36616	36247	31636	58724	07206
98383	08409	04051	55470	38757	89765	41036	09538
89346	90068	17162	56999	61095	83147	40757	58153
56017	37731	08626	08157	19292	32275	93574	32589
91202	58841	59745	98489	59264	44396	68511	07135

APPENDIX C

RANDOM ALLOCATION OF TREATMENTS TO INDIVIDUAL SURVEY UNITS (VILLAGES, ETC.) OR EXPERIMENTAL SUBJECTS (PATIENTS, ETC.) BEARING SERIAL NUMBERS

Serial number of the experimental or survey unit	Allocation to treatment group (A,B,C, etc.) when the total number of treatments experimented upon is:								
	2	3	4	5	6	7	8	9	10
1	B	A	C	C	B	E	F	A	J
2	A	B	A	B	C	D	G	C	C
3	A	A	C	E	F	D	E	H	B
4	B	C	D	B	A	F	D	F	A
5	A	A	B	C	D	C	A	E	D
6	B	B	A	D	E	B	C	D	G
7	B	C	C	B	B	B	B	B	I
8	A	A	D	D	A	A	A	C	C
9	A	C	B	E	D	G	H	B	A
10	A	B	A	A	F	C	E	H	F
11	A	B	D	A	A	D	E	D	E
12	B	C	A	E	C	E	F	G	G
13	B	C	B	D	E	A	B	E	I
14	A	A	D	C	B	G	D	I	J
15	B	B	A	A	F	F	H	I	B
16	A	C	B	C	A	B	A	A	E
17	A	B	C	E	A	G	E	F	H
18	B	B	D	B	C	C	D	C	A
19	A	A	B	C	B	F	G	H	J
20	B	A	C	D	C	E	C	B	D
21	A	C	D	A	D	D	F	I	B
22	B	B	A	D	E	G	A	G	D
23	A	A	B	E	D	C	G	B	F
24	B	B	B	A	F	B	D	D	A
25	B	C	D	B	C	A	H	A	H

Appendix C

Serial number of the experimental or survey unit	Allocation to treatment group (A,B,C, etc.) when the total number of treatments experimented upon is:								
	2	3	4	5	6	7	8	9	10
26	A	C	A	E	E	E	B	F	E
27	B	A	D	D	A	F	C	C	G
28	B	B	C	D	B	C	H	E	H
29	B	C	C	D	D	A	F	I	B
30	B	A	C	B	F	D	F	A	I
31	A	B	C	C	E	G	G	F	J
32	A	B	B	C	E	E	B	G	F
33	B	C	A	E	F	A	C	D	C
34	B	A	D	A	A	F	H	H	H
35	B	A	D	E	F	B	E	E	D
36	A	C	B	A	A	E	C	G	F
37	B	A	A	E	D	C	A	A	C
38	A	A	C	B	C	G	D	F	G
39	A	B	C	D	C	B	G	B	I
40	B	B	B	C	C	E	B	I	E
41	B	C	A	C	F	A	H	E	B
42	A	A	D	E	C	E	E	C	H
43	B	B	B	A	B	C	A	I	F
44	B	C	C	D	F	B	D	H	J
45	A	C	D	C	C	D	C	D	A
46	A	B	B	E	E	F	E	B	J
47	B	A	A	B	B	D	G	G	F
48	B	A	D	C	E	G	H	H	G
49	B	C	B	E	F	B	F	D	H
50	A	A	A	C	A	D	D	F	B
51	B	B	A	D	B	F	E	B	C
52	A	B	C	E	C	C	C	H	J
53	B	A	B	A	A	G	C	E	A
54	B	B	C	D	F	C	F	E	B
55	A	A	D	D	F	B	D	H	E

Appendix C

Serial number of the experimental or survey unit	Allocation to treatment group (A,B,C, etc.) when the total number of treatments experimented upon is:								
	2	3	4	5	6	7	8	9	10
56	B	B	C	E	E	E	G	F	B
57	A	B	C	B	A	B	A	G	A
58	B	C	A	D	E	C	G	D	H
59	B	B	A	C	C	B	B	F	C
60	B	A	D	C	F	D	F	D	I
61	A	A	D	D	F	C	D	A	B
62	A	B	C	B	E	A	E	I	A
63	B	C	B	A	B	C	F	H	H
64	B	A	A	A	D	B	F	E	H
65	A	A	D	C	C	F	H	E	J
66	B	C	B	E	F	B	C	I	F
67	A	C	C	D	C	G	E	H	E
68	B	B	C	C	C	E	D	G	C
69	B	B	C	B	F	D	F	H	E
70	A	C	A	E	D	A	C	F	A
71	A	A	B	C	C	D	C	G	E
72	B	B	D	A	E	G	B	D	E
73	B	A	A	B	D	E	B	I	D
74	B	A	B	E	A	F	H	I	H
75	A	A	A	A	E	B	E	B	D
76	B	B	A	D	D	D	E	H	F
77	A	B	B	C	C	A	D	A	I
78	A	C	B	A	B	D	F	C	B
79	B	C	D	A	C	B	G	G	I
80	A	B	A	B	F	F	C	I	C
81	A	A	D	E	C	E	A	E	I
82	B	A	C	B	C	A	C	G	G
83	A	C	C	D	A	C	A	D	H
84	B	A	B	E	B	E	F	I	E
85	A	A	A	C	C	G	C	B	C

Serial number of the experimental or survey unit	Allocation to treatment group (A,B,C, etc.) when the total number of treatments experimented upon is:								
	2	3	4	5	6	7	8	9	10
86	B	B	B	D	A	C	A	F	G
87	A	C	A	D	C	A	H	F	I
88	A	B	D	D	B	F	C	C	I
89	A	C	C	C	F	B	G	E	E
90	B	B	B	A	D	D	D	A	B
91	B	C	C	D	E	F	C	E	J
92	A	B	D	B	C	E	D	G	B
93	B	C	C	A	A	G	B	C	B
94	A	A	B	B	E	A	G	B	G
95	B	A	B	C	A	C	E	A	C
96	B	B	A	B	D	E	G	D	H
97	A	B	B	E	A	A	G	B	I
98	B	A	C	B	C	G	A	G	I
99	A	C	A	B	F	C	E	A	E
100	B	A	D	D	B	D	H	B	C
101	B	B	A	D	E	E	D	C	B
102	B	C	D	A	A	F	B	B	J
103	B	B	C	C	C	A	C	G	J
104	A	C	C	D	D	A	F	B	C
105	A	B	A	C	F	D	G	A	D
106	B	C	B	B	A	F	C	D	E
107	A	A	D	C	F	D	G	G	H
108	B	A	B	B	D	D	B	C	A
109	A	A	C	B	A	A	F	F	J
110	B	C	C	E	B	A	E	D	J
111	A	C	A	A	E	B	A	I	G
112	A	A	C	E	B	F	A	G	J
113	A	C	D	A	C	G	F	C	G
114	B	B	C	C	D	A	D	B	E
115	A	C	B	B	F	E	H	B	F

Appendix C

Serial number of the experimental or survey unit	Allocation to treatment group (A,B,C, etc.) when the total number of treatments experimented upon is:								
	2	3	4	5	6	7	8	9	10
116	A	C	D	E	A	B	B	C	J
117	A	A	D	C	E	E	E	A	H
118	B	A	B	D	C	C	H	C	C
119	A	B	D	B	D	F	H	F	J
120	A	B	C	A	F	C	A	D	F
121	A	B	D	C	E	E	C	I	A
122	B	C	B	B	A	B	E	H	I
123	A	C	C	E	E	F	H	C	I
124	A	A	C	B	B	B	A	G	I
125	B	B	A	E	D	F	H	F	G
126	A	A	A	C	D	B	E	C	F
127	A	A	C	B	A	G	F	A	C
128	A	C	B	D	B	C	B	H	E
129	B	C	C	A	A	A	A	E	D
130	A	A	A	E	E	C	D	E	D
131	B	B	B	A	B	C	A	D	E
132	A	C	D	B	A	D	E	I	J
133	A	A	C	E	D	E	B	F	F
134	B	B	A	E	E	A	H	G	I
135	A	A	C	C	D	G	B	B	G
136	B	A	B	B	A	G	G	F	C
137	A	B	A	E	B	D	B	A	C
138	A	C	D	A	E	E	D	H	A
139	B	A	B	C	A	C	E	D	I
140	A	C	A	B	C	D	G	F	I
141	B	B	D	C	B	B	C	E	D
142	A	C	B	E	B	A	A	I	H
143	B	C	D	C	D	C	H	D	F
144	B	B	A	D	F	F	E	F	D
145	A	C	B	D	B	G	B	E	D

Serial number of the experimental or survey unit	Allocation to treatment group (A,B,C, etc.) when the total number of treatments experimented upon is:								
	2	3	4	5	6	7	8	9	10
146	B	A	A	A	C	A	H	I	E
147	A	C	C	D	F	F	D	E	F
148	B	B	B	C	A	E	G	I	D
149	A	C	A	D	E	A	F	C	F
150	A	A	C	A	F	F	G	H	D
151	B	C	A	A	F	G	H	C	C
152	A	A	D	A	C	G	E	F	J
153	A	B	B	D	E	B	F	G	H
154	A	B	B	A	B	E	C	E	G
155	A	A	C	E	E	A	G	D	B
156	B	B	C	D	D	A	C	F	H
157	A	A	B	E	B	E	D	D	E
158	A	B	C	C	D	E	G	D	D
159	B	A	A	B	A	E	B	C	C
160	B	B	B	E	F	B	A	C	I
161	A	C	B	D	C	G	B	B	A
162	A	C	D	B	A	B	G	C	B
163	A	B	D	A	B	E	H	G	E
164	B	B	A	E	A	C	A	A	F
165	B	C	B	A	D	D	B	H	A
166	B	B	D	C	E	F	F	D	I
167	B	A	D	A	A	C	E	E	G
168	A	B	C	D	D	G	A	F	A
169	B	A	A	E	E	E	D	D	H
170	A	C	C	A	D	D	G	D	C
171	B	C	A	D	E	G	E	G	D
172	B	A	D	B	F	G	C	B	H
173	B	B	A	E	E	D	H	A	B
174	A	A	C	C	C	A	B	I	C
175	B	C	B	A	A	E	D	A	D

Appendix C

Serial number of the experimental or survey unit.	Allocation of treatment group (A,B,C, etc.) when the total number of treatments experimented upon is:								
	2	3	4	5	6	7	8	9	10
176	B	C	D	E	F	A	C	D	C
177	A	A	C	B	B	G	F	F	I
178	A	C	C	A	C	C	G	B	G
179	B	B	B	B	F	B	H	H	E
180	B	B	A	C	A	F	G	H	G
181	A	A	D	D	E	G	E	F	H
182	B	B	A	A	A	G	H	A	J
183	A	A	C	D	C	A	D	I	F
184	D	C	B	B	D	B	B	H	D
185	A	A	D	E	F	C	C	C	F
186	A	A	D	D	B	D	D	E	H
187	B	C	D	D	C	A	A	B	E
188	B	A	C	B	D	F	A	D	I
189	A	B	B	C	A	D	B	G	C
190	A	A	A	D	A	A	G	H	B
191	B	C	B	E	F	D	H	C	J
192	A	B	D	A	B	E	B	F	F
193	B	C	B	E	E	D	E	H	F
194	B	B	A	D	C	F	D	B	A
195	A	A	C	D	D	D	F	A	A
196	B	C	D	C	E	F	A	I	A
197	B	C	C	A	F	B	D	C	J
198	A	C	D	C	D	B	H	E	J
199	A	A	D	B	B	G	C	A	I
200	B	C	A	E	C	C	B	C	E

APPENDIX D

TABLE of X^2 at 5% and 1% levels of significance

Degree of Freedom n	P = .05	P = .01
1	3.841	6.635
2	5.991	9.210
3	7.815	11.345
4	9.488	13.277
5	11,070	15,086
6	12.592	16.812
7	14.067	18.475
8	15.507	20.090
9	16.919	21.666
10	18.307	23.209
11	19.675	24.725
12	21.026	26.217
13	22.362	27.688
14	23.685	29.141
15	24,996	30.578
16	26.296	32.000
17	27.587	33.409
18	28.869	34.805
19	30.144	36.191
20	31,410	37,566
21	32.671	38.932
22	33.924	40.289
23	35.172	41.638
24	36.415	42.980
25	37,652	44,314
26	38.885	45.642
27	40.113	46.963
28	41.337	48.278
29	42.557	49.588
30	43.773	50.892

Note: If the degrees of freedom are more than 30, use the following method:

Calculate $\sqrt{2 X^2} - \sqrt{2n - 1}$

If this quantity exceeds 2.33, X^2 is significant at 1% (P = .01) probability level. If this quantity exceeds 1.64, X^2 is significant at 5% (P = .05) probability level.

Source: R.A. Fisher and F. Yates, Statistical tables for biological agricultural and medical research (1953) table IV

APPENDIX E

Table of "t" at 5% and 1% levels of significance

Degrees of freedom n	P = .05	P = .01
1	12.706	63.657
2	4.303	9.925
3	3.182	5.841
4	2.776	4.604
5	2.571	4.032
6	2.447	3.707
7	2.365	3.499
8	2.306	3.355
9	2.262	3.250
10	2.228	3.169
11	2.201	3.106
12	2.179	3.055
13	2.160	3.012
14	2.145	2.977
15	2.131	2.947
16	2.120	2.921
17	2.110	2.898
18	2.101	2.878
19	2.093	2.861
20	2.086	2.845
21	2.080	2.831
22	2.074	2.819
23	2.069	2.807
24	2.064	2.797
25	2.060	2.787
26	2.056	2.779
27	2.052	2.771
28	2.048	2.763
29	2.045	2.756
30	2.042	2.750
40	2.021	2.704
60	2.000	2.660
120	1.980	2.617
∞	1.960	2.576

Source: R.A. Fisher and F. Yates, Statistical Tables for Biological, Agricultural and Medical Research (1953) table V.

REFERENCES

Archibald, H. M. & Bruce-Chwatt, L. J. (1956) Suppression of malaria with pyrimethamine in Nigerian school children, Bull. Wld Hlth Org. 15, 775-784

Barber, M. A. & Mayne, B. (1924) The seasonal incidence of types of malaria parasites in the Southern United States, Sth. med. J. (Bgham, Ala.), 17, 583

Boyd, M. F. (1949) Malariology, vols I and II, Philadelphia

Bruce-Chwatt, L. J. (1956) Biometric study of spleen and liver weights in Africans and Europeans with special reference to endemic malaria, Bull. Wld Hlth Org. 15, No. 3-5, pp. 513-548

Casey, R. S. & Perry, J. W. (1951) Punched cards - their application to science and industry, New York

Ceylon (1935) Supplement to the Sessional Paper XXII. The Ceylon malaria epidemic 1934-1935, Ceylon Government Press, Colombo

Cochran, W. G. & Cox, G. M. (1950) Experimental designs, New York

Covell, G., Russell, P. F. & Swellengrabel, N. H. (1953) Malaria terminology, Report of a drafting committee appointed by the World Health Organization, Geneva

Dakshinamurty, S. (1948) Measurement of malaria, Part II, Indian J. Malar. 2, 129-156

Eisenhart, C., Hastay, M. W. & Wallis, W. A. (1947) Selected techniques of statistical analysis, New York

Finney, D. J. (1952) Probit analysis. A statistical treatment of the sigmoid response curve, 2nd ed., Cambridge University Press

Fisher, R. A. (1950) Statistical methods for research workers, 11th ed., Edinburgh

Fisher, R. A. (1951) The design of experiments, 6th ed., Edinburgh

Fisher, R. A. & Yates, F. (1953) Statistical tables for biological, agricultural and medical research, 4th ed., Edinburgh

Gabaldon, A. (1949) The nationwide campaign against malaria in Venezuela, Trans. roy. Soc. trop. Med. Hyg. 43, 113-164

Gabaldon, A. (1956) The time required to reach eradication in relation to malaria constitution, Amer. J. trop. Med. Hyg. 5, No. 6, pp. 966-976

Gill, C. A. (1928) The genesis of epidemics and the natural history of disease, London

Gunaratna, L. F. (1956) Recent antimalaria work in Ceylon, Bull. Wld Hlth Org. 15, No. 3-5, p. 796

Hald, A. (1952) Statistical tables and formulas, New York

Hill, B. (1955) Principles of medical statistics, 6th ed., Lancet

Hill, R. N., Cambournac, F. J. C. & Simoes, M. P. (1943) Observations on the course of malaria in children in an endemic region, Amer. J. trop. Med. 23, 147

Howard, E. C., Earle, W. C. & Muench, H. (1935) A method of analysis of field malaria data, J. Amer. statist. Ass. 30, 249-256

Iyengar, M. O. T. (1932) Seasonal incidence of tertian, subtertian and quartan infections, Indian J. med. Res. 20, 303

Joncour, G. (1956) La lutte contre la paludisme à Madagascar, Bull. Wld Hlth Org. 15, 711-723

Litchfield, J. T. & Wilcoxon, F. (1949) J. Pharmacol. 95, 99

Macchiavello, A. (1955) Principles of project evaluation, (Unpublished working document WHO/VDT/150)

Macdonald, G. (1955) A new approach to the epidemiology of malaria, Indian J. Malar, 9 4, 261

MacDonald, G. (1956) Theory of eradication of malaria, Bull. Wld Hlth Org. 15, 369-387

Mainland, D. (1952) Elementary medical statistics, Philadelphia

Mayne, B. (1928) The influence of relative humidity on the presence of parasites in the insect carrier and the initial seasonal appearance of malaria in a selected area in India, Indian J. med. Res. 15, 1073

Molina, G. & Puffer, R. R. (1955) Informe sobre las condiciones sanitaries en las Americas, 1950-1953, Bol. Ofic. sanit. pan-amer. 39, 331

Pampana, E. J. (1954) Effect of malaria control on birth and death rates, Proceedings of the World Population Conference, Rome, United Nations Document E/Conf. 13/413, pp. 497-510

Pampana, E. J. (1955) Some malaria eradication problems as visualized in 1955, Indian J. Malar. 9, 4, pp. 361-369

Pletsch, D. J. & Ch'en, C. T. (1954) Economic and social effects of malaria control with some specific instances from Taiwan (Unpublished working document WHO/Mal/108)

Pryde, J., ed. (1948) Chamber's seven-figure mathematical tables, London

Rajinda Pal (1945) On the bionomics of Anopheles culicifacies Giles, Part IV, J. Malar. Inst. India, 6, 239-241

Ross, R. & Stott, W. (1911) Tables of statistical error, Ann. trop. Med. Parasit. 5, 347-369

Ross, R. (1916) Proc. roy. Soc. Ser. A, 92, 204

Russell, P. F., West, L. S. & Manwell, R. D. (1946) Practical malariology, Philadelphia

Schuffner, W. A. P. (1938) J. Malar. Inst. India, 1, 221

Snedecor, G. W. (1956) Statistical methods allied to experiments in agriculture and biology, 5th ed. Iowa State College Press, Ames, Iowa

Swaroop, S. (1957) Index of endemicity, Bull. Wld Hlth Org. 16, No. 6, p. 1083

United Nations (1950) The preparation of sampling survey reports, United Nations Statistical Papers, Series C, No. 1, Rev.

United Nations (1952) Demographic year book, 1952, New York

United Nations (1953) Principles for a vital statistics system. Recommendations for the improvement and standardization of vital statistics. Statistical Papers, Series M, No. 19, New York

United Nations (1955) Statistical sampling. International recommendations and developments concerning their application. (Working document Group IV, Proceedings III Inter-American Statistical Conference, Quitandinha, Brazil)

USA (1954) On the use of sampling in the field of public health. Committee on sampling techniques in public health statistics, Amer. J. publ. Hlth, 44, 719-740

Viswanathan, D. K., Ramachandra Ras T., & Bhatia, S. C. (1952) The validity of estimation of anopheles densities on the basis of hand collection on a timed basis from fixed catching stations. Indian J. Malar. 6, 2, pp. 199-213

Wenyon, C. M. (1921) The incidence and aetiology of malaria in Macedonia, 1915-1919, J. roy. Army med. Cps, 37, 172, 264, 352

World Health Organization (1957) Manual of the International Statistical Classification of Diseases, Injuries, and Causes of Death, Geneva, 2 vols (1955 Revision)

World Health Organization, Expert Committee on Health Statistics (1950) Report of the second session, Wld Hlth Org. techn. Rep. Ser. 25

World Health Organization, Expert Committee on Malaria (1950b) Report of the third session, Wld Hlth Org. techn. Rep. Ser. 8, 15

World Health Organization, Expert Committee on Malaria (1951) Report of the fourth session, Wld Hlth Org. techn. Rep. Ser. 39

World Health Organization (1951b) Report of the malaria conference in Equatorial Africa, Wld Hlth Org. techn. Rep. Ser. 38, 45

World Health Organization (1953) Epidem. vital. Statist. Rep. Part I & II

World Health Organization (1954) Off. Rec. Wld Hlth Org. 52, 35-52

World Health Organization (1955) Off. Rec. Wld Hlth Org. 60, 33-45

World Health Organization (1956a) Malaria Conference for the Western Pacific and
    South-East Asia Regions. Second Asian Malaria Conference, Baguio, Philippines,
    November 1954, Wld Hlth Org. techn. Rep. Ser. 103

World Health Organization, Expert Committee on Malaria (1956b) Sixth Report
    (Unpublished working document WHO/Mal/180)

Yacob, M. & Swaroop, S. (1945) Investigation of long-term periodicity in the
    incidence of epidemic malaria in the Punjab, J. Malar. Inst. India, 6, 39-51

Yacob, M. & Swaroop, S. (1947) Malaria and spleen rate in the Punjab,
    Indian J. Malar. 469-501

Yates, F. (1953) Sampling methods for censuses and surveys, 2nd ed., London